Planning Parenthood

Planning Parenthood

Strategies for Success in Fertility Assistance,
Adoption, and Surrogacy

Rebecca A. Clark, M.D., Ph.D.

Gloria Richard-Davis, M.D., FACOG

Jill Hayes, Ph.D.

Michelle Murphy, J.D.

Katherine Pucheu Theall, Ph.D.

THE JOHNS HOPKINS UNIVERSITY PRESS

BALTIMORE

Note to the reader: This book is not intended to provide medical or legal advice. The services of a competent professional should be obtained whenever medical, legal, or other specific advice is needed.

© 2009 The Johns Hopkins University Press
All rights reserved. Published 2009
Printed in the United States of America on acid-free paper
9 8 7 6 5 4 3 2 1

The Johns Hopkins University Press
2715 North Charles Street
Baltimore, Maryland 21218-4363
www.press.jhu.edu

Library of Congress Cataloging-in-Publication Data

Planning parenthood : strategies for success in fertility assistance, adoption, and surrogacy / Rebecca A. Clark . . . [et al.].
    p. cm.
   Includes bibliographical references and index.
   ISBN-13: 978-0-8018-9111-3 (hardcover : alk. paper)
   ISBN-10: 0-8018-9111-6 (hardcover : alk. paper)
   ISBN-13: 978-0-8018-9112-0 (pbk. : alk. paper)
   ISBN-10: 0-8018-9112-4 (pbk. : alk. paper)
   1. Human reproductive technology—Popular works.   2. Surrogate motherhood.
3. Infertility—Popular works.   4. Adoption.   I. Clark, Rebecca A., 1958–
RG133.5.P618   2009
618.1'78—dc22   2008023838

A catalog record for this book is available from the British Library.

Special discounts are available for bulk purchases of this book. For more information, please contact Special Sales at 410-516-6936 or specialsales@press.jhu.edu.

The Johns Hopkins University Press uses environmentally friendly book materials, including recycled text paper that is composed of at least 30 percent post-consumer waste, whenever possible. All of our book papers are acid-free, and our jackets and covers are printed on paper with recycled content.

CONTENTS

PREFACE

About This Book

Raising a child is one of the most rewarding things a person can do, and most people reach a point in their lives when they decide, consciously or not, that they want to be a parent. For a very large number of women and men, though, becoming a parent is not as easy as tossing away the birth control and welcoming a baby into the world nine months later. In fact, every year, hundreds of thousands of American couples are unable to conceive and they seek fertility advice. Many other individuals have limited options for achieving parenthood because they are single or older or in a same-sex relationship. Other people have a medical condition or an inheritable disease that restricts how they become parents.

Fertility assistance, surrogacy, and adoption help people overcome these hurdles and become parents. Within each of these pathways to parenthood are further categories: minimally invasive fertility assistance methods and more invasive assisted reproduction techniques; traditional surrogacy and gestational surrogacy; and public, private, and independent domestic adoptions and international adoptions. Deciding which pathway to follow can be mind-boggling, to say the least. Factors such as a woman's age, an individual's genetic history, or a couple's living situation can all play a part in the decision.

We are five professionals—two physicians, a psychologist, an epidemiologist, and a lawyer—who decided to compile our professional experience and write a book that provides the basic information that people need to know about each option for achieving parenthood so that they can decide which pathway will work best for them. Some of us are also parents who have struggled in our own ways to achieve parenthood. During the process we considered the pros and cons of our various options by scouring the available literature and asking our friends for advice. We found the search for data to be challenging, since there wasn't one source that compared critical information about each pathway. The "conception" of this book resulted from the frustration we felt. We have done our best to lay out what you need to know to make an informed decision about your strategy to become a parent.

This book gives you an overview of what you can anticipate from the various pathways to parenthood. Some people may view the options as steps along a continuum, starting with minimal fertility assistance and proceeding through every intervention shown in figure P.1 before finally moving to adoption. Although fertility assistance can be thought of as consisting of various stages with obvious stopping points, not everyone needs to go through every step. You may decide to stop at a certain point and pursue adoption. Some people may start at the "other options" category shown at the bottom of the figure because, for example, a woman has already gone through menopause or a gay couple is interested in pursuing surrogacy. In the first half of the book, we describe what's involved in each option for becoming a parent.

We hope that this book will help you decide on a strategy before you embark on any pathway to parenthood. We suggest that you set goals for when to stop pursuing one option and switch to another; doing so will make it easier to accept that you aren't having success on that pathway and you need to move to another. This book can help you to outline a plan that you can afford financially and emotionally and that poses risks you feel comfortable with. We want you to weigh the pros and cons of the options available to you. The primary "pro" for all options is becoming a parent. The main differences between pathways are the "cons" in getting there, such as medical and emotional risks and time, hassle, and financial costs. In the second half of the book, we concentrate predominantly on these cons, although we also note positive aspects that are worth considering. We want you to be well informed about the risks but not discouraged by them.

We review fertility assistance methods (including donor sperm, eggs, and embryos), surrogacy, and adoption (domestic and international) as possible pathways to parenthood. In part I, the first seven chapters describe what to expect with each option. Two

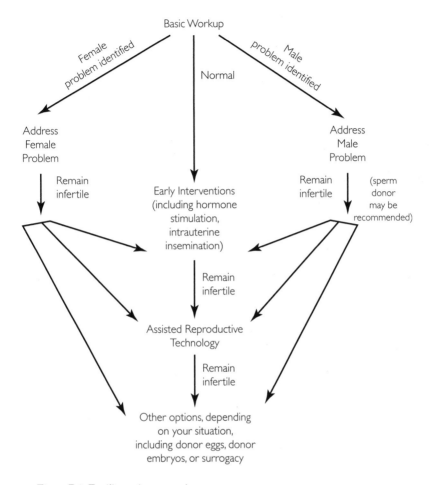

Figure P.1. Fertility assistance options.

additional chapters discuss the requirements for each option and considerations for nontraditional families. The chapters in part II compare the options and identify potential risks and costs (medical, mental health, emotional, time, "hassle," and financial) and legal considerations for each option. At the end of each chapter, we include a personal story—some of these are our stories, some are stories of our patients and acquaintances. Contributors were asked to share their experiences or one aspect of their experience that they would want others to know about. Both positive and negative points that may not be apparent in the body of the chapters are illustrated in these stories.

Once you choose the pathway you wish to take, you should do additional research. At the end of the text in each we list several excellent references and internet sources to help you continue your research. If you are interested in detailed scientific papers on various subjects, you may want to consult the list of references that we consulted in writing the chapters. These references appear at the end of the book. We also include a glossary of terms and appendixes that summarize the major considerations for each option.

As you read, keep in mind that almost any person who is a loving individual and who can provide a safe home is able to become a parent. To get there, however, requires persistence, time, and dedication. At the moment it may seem that it will take forever to become a parent. Fortunately, the journey to becoming a parent is time-limited. Most people bring home a baby or child within two years of beginning the journey along one of the pathways described in this book. For many, it will take even less time—a matter of months to a year. The financial costs can be daunting. In the grand scheme of things, though, the financial costs of becoming a parent (not including the costs of being a parent) are generally only a fraction of your lifetime earnings. By surmounting the barriers you face in making your family, you are demonstrating your commitment and readiness for parenthood. The highs you will experience as a parent are probably going to be proportional to the lows you experience on the journey to get there.

Remember, too, that you are far from alone in seeking fertility assistance, surrogacy, or adoption to have children. About 15 percent of the sixty million American women of reproductive age have received fertility treatment at some point in their lives. Every year, more than one million American couples seek medical advice or treatment for infertility. In 2005, the most recent year with available data, 52,041 babies were born in the United States as a result of assisted reproductive technologies. Every year in the United

States, more than 120,000 children are adopted, about 90 percent of them domestically and 10 percent internationally.

Virtually everyone who wants to be a parent can be. The only real criteria are being flexible and being ready to invest some time, money, and energy into achieving the dream. We hope this book will be helpful as you decide how you want to proceed, and we wholeheartedly wish you success on your journey to becoming a parent.

PART I

What Are the Pathways to Parenthood?

Many options are available for women, men, and couples wanting a child. When you decide to seek assistance to have a child, you want to have some idea of what these options are and what is involved for each one. In this section, we describe fertility assessment tests, assisted reproduction techniques, and adoption pathways. By understanding what each of these pathways entails, you can weigh your options and decide which pathway or pathways will best suit your circumstances and desires.

Chapter 1

THE FERTILITY WORKUP

Starting the fertility workup is exciting. You may quickly find out what your problem is, and it may be a problem that is easily treated. Or it may take some time to identify the problem. In either case, you are taking the next steps to achieve parenthood. You can feel good about taking control and you can be optimistic about the future.

Here's what you can expect during the initial fertility workup, which often takes several weeks to complete:

- The person who examines you (usually a physician) will take a basic medical history and perform a physical examination, including, for women, a pelvic examination.
- You will undergo a series of relatively simple, inexpensive tests, usually including, for women, a Pap smear, testing for sexually transmitted infections, and blood tests, and, for men, a sperm analysis and blood tests. The blood tests ordered for the fertility workup check selected hormone levels to determine whether you are ovulating, are close to menopause, or have an underlying condition such as an underactive or overactive thyroid. Several immune disorders can cause fertility problems, so you may be tested for these disorders via blood tests.
- A method to determine the woman's ovulation pattern is initiated. Methods for checking ovulation can include the no-cost, old-fashioned basal temperature monitoring or

newer ovulation prediction tests, which use urine or saliva to check for ovulation.

- The postcoital test is sometimes done. The couple is asked to have intercourse around the time of ovulation, and then, approximately 4 to 12 hours later, a sample of mucus is taken from the woman's cervix. Your doctor can check how well the sperm function in the vaginal environment by looking at the mucus specimen under a microscope. If the doctor suspects a problem with how the sperm are able to function in the vagina, then he or she may recommend that the sperm be inserted directly into the uterus (thus bypassing the vaginal environment). This method of insemination is called intrauterine insemination (IUI) and is described in the next chapter.

- A test that is usually performed in women over the age of thirty-five years is the Clomid challenge test. Clomid or Serophene (brand names), or clomiphene citrate (generic name), is a medication that stimulates egg production. The Clomid challenge test indicates whether the woman has adequate "ovarian reserve" (has a sufficient number of eggs) and whether her eggs are viable (healthy and able to be fertilized and produce a baby). As we emphasize in many places in this book, the chance of a woman having a successful pregnancy with her own eggs depends greatly on her age. As a woman approaches age forty, the chances of a successful pregnancy outcome with her own eggs rapidly diminish. In the Clomid challenge test, the woman's hormone levels (estrogen and follicle-stimulating hormone) are checked on about day 3 of the menstrual cycle, she takes the Clomid, and then these hormone levels are rechecked. The estrogen or estradiol level should rise by the fifth day, but if the woman's follicle-stimulating hormone (FSH) level is elevated on either day 2 or after five days, she very likely does not have adequate ovarian reserve. Although she is unlikely to be able to become pregnant with her own eggs, donor eggs may be a good option.

HYSTEROSALPINGOGRAM AND LAPAROSCOPY

After you undergo the basic workup, your doctor may recommend additional tests.

Women who have a blockage in their fallopian tube or tubes have more difficulty becoming pregnant; if both tubes are completely blocked, she may not be able to conceive through intercourse or insemination. If the basic workup does not reveal a reason for infertility, the physician will probably recommend a hysterosalpingogram (HSG). In this test, dye is injected into the uterus and fallopian tubes, and then X-rays are taken. The radiologist can determine whether there are blockages in the tubes and whether there is any other reason that may be keeping the woman from getting pregnant. HSGs can be uncomfortable, causing mild to severe cramping for a few hours after the procedure. If your tubes are slightly blocked, the doctor may push the dye more forcefully to try to clear the block, and this maneuver can increase the cramping. Generally the woman can return to work the same day.

A second test that may be done either early or late in the workup is a laparoscopy. This surgical procedure is done as an outpatient surgery and requires anesthesia. A laparoscopy involves placing a lighted telescope and other instruments through a small cut (less than one inch) in the abdomen. The doctor can then see any abnormalities of the uterus and surrounding area, such as endometriosis. Endometriosis is a disorder in which tissue normally found in the uterus (called endometrial tissue) is located in various places in the pelvic area. Endometriosis can be both diagnosed and treated during a laparoscopy. Scar tissue can also be removed during the procedure. The most common problems following laparoscopy are pain around the cut or discomfort in the right shoulder from the carbon dioxide used to inflate the abdomen. After the procedure, women generally feel well enough to go back to normal activities within one or two days.

WHAT HAPPENS AFTER THE FERTILITY WORKUP?

Your doctor will discuss the findings from the basic workup with you and recommend what to do next. If your infertility is not explained by any of the test results, you probably will be offered early fertility assistance, as described in the next chapter. You may also decide not to pursue fertility assistance at this point and, instead, proceed to adoption choices.

FURTHER READING

J. Meyers-Thompson and S. Perkins. *Fertility for Dummies.* Wiley, 2003.

WHEN I WAS THIRTY, my husband and I decided to start a family. Because my mother and sister had conceived in the very month they planned to, I assumed the same would happen for me. It didn't, and month after month went by. After 10 months, I went to see my family doctor, who said I should keep trying for another few months and then come back. I did, and she told me I was young and healthy and should give it another 3 months. Three months later she said the same thing, and I started feeling really frustrated. Still, I followed her advice. When more than a year and a half had gone by, I finally came to my senses and found a new doctor.

My new doctor did a fertility workup on me, including a hysterosalpingogram, which felt as if my insides were being pinched. She also had my husband's sperm tested. Everything was normal with our test results. The diagnosis of unexplained infertility was frustrating in itself, because we had nothing concrete to try to fix. My doctor recommended that I take Clomid, so I did, with progesterone supplementation, for seven consecutive months. On the seventh month I conceived. My husband and I were thrilled! The first trimester went well and I felt great. At 12 weeks gestation, my doctor was unable to find a heartbeat with the Doppler, so she scheduled an ultrasound. I was nervous going to the appointment, but all was well and I saw our little baby waving its arms and legs and sipping amniotic fluid. At 16 weeks, my doctor again couldn't find the heartbeat and I went for another ultrasound, excited at the prospect of seeing the baby again. My husband came too. This time, though, there was no heartbeat. We were stunned. We had thought that everything would be fine once we got through the first trimester. I was admitted into the hospital and induced into labor. We were devastated to suddenly find ourselves back at square one.

We couldn't bear the thought of going back on Clomid, especially since I had only 5 months left of the 12-month lifetime maximum my doctor was willing to give me. Instead, she referred us to a fertility clinic, where we began hormone stimulation treatments with IUI. We had to travel four hours by car to the fertility clinic, so it was difficult to schedule the treatment. In the end, I stayed with friends to take the hormones and my husband traveled to meet me once I knew when the IUI was scheduled. After the initial apprehension of jabbing a needle in my own belly every day, I was glad to be doing the hormone stimulation. I felt as if I had gained a little bit of control and was doing something positive toward our goal of having a baby. I was excited when, after nine days of injections and blood tests, the nurse sent me for an ultrasound. I had four large follicles and several smaller ones. That night I injected the hormone to induce me to ovulate, and my husband arrived to give his sperm sample the next morning. He was worried about freezing up when he had to perform, because the timing was tight to get as fresh a sample as possible to the clinic. But he didn't, and we drove the 15 minutes to the clinic, arriving exactly two hours before the scheduled IUI so that the lab could wash and prepare the sperm sample. The IUI itself was practically a non-event: the nurse inserted the sperm with a catheter and I then lay quietly for half an hour thinking about the baby we were about to conceive and worrying a little about conceiving multiples. Two weeks later, the pregnancy test was negative. I was crushed.

We skipped a month and then repeated the procedure. This second attempt was also unsuccessful, but somehow it didn't hurt me emotionally as much as the negative result after the first attempt. The clinic's policy was to meet with patients after two unsuccessful treatments to discuss next steps. Our fertility specialist reviewed our history and suggested that we could continue with hormone stimulation and IUI or move on to try IVF (in vitro fertilization). At this point, it was late September and we were worn out from the two unsuccessful IUIs and all the traveling back and forth. We opted to take a break for the rest of the year and to try an IVF cycle the following January.

As fate would have it, we conceived with no outside assistance in October. This unexpected pregnancy progressed normally, and at 38 weeks I delivered a beautiful, healthy baby girl. Our daughter is now seven months old and an absolute delight. I still get the shivers when I think of everything we went through to become parents, and I wonder if we'll be able to have a second child. But for now, we're simply savoring life as a family of three.

Chapter 2

EARLY FERTILITY ASSISTANCE

Hormone Stimulation and
Intrauterine Insemination

We hope the reason for your infertility is apparent from the basic workup so that your doctor can recommend specific next steps. Unfortunately, for many women the initial test results do not explain why they are having difficulty conceiving. In this case, the doctor will probably suggest using medications to improve the woman's chances of ovulating and conceiving.

HORMONE STIMULATION

Clomid (the medication used in the challenge test mentioned in chapter 1) is one of the first medications tried for hormone stimulation, particularly if a woman does not ovulate or if the length of her menstrual cycle varies from month to month. Clomid, which is taken as a pill, stimulates the ovaries to make and release an egg or several eggs and to provide better hormonal support to achieve pregnancy. Approximately four out of five women will ovulate in response to the stimulation of follicle-stimulating hormone (FSH) by Clomid.

Potential risks from taking Clomid include multiple births, which occur in 5 to 10 percent of Clomid cycles, and, rarely, over-

stimulating the ovaries. Overstimulation, often called ovarian hyperstimulation, occurs when a woman's estrogen levels become excessively high. Both of these complications are discussed in more
depth in chapter 11. Possible side effects while taking Clomid include hot flashes, headaches, nausea, and blurred vision; some
women report several of these symptoms and others experience
none of them. The American Society for Reproductive Medicine
recommends that a woman take no more than six cycles of Clomid during her lifetime, once ovulation is achieved. For a woman
over thirty-five years of age, it is generally not worth persevering
with Clomid if she does not conceive in the first few cycles. (A
Clomid cycle is like a woman's regular monthly cycle but may be
longer between periods.)

If a woman does not conceive on Clomid cycles, her doctor may
recommend trying injectable hormones to stimulate egg production. Injecting hormones to increase the number of eggs or to mature the eggs is called controlled ovarian hyperstimulation. We refer to this process throughout the book as hormone stimulation.
The goal of hormone stimulation is to instruct the ovaries to make
and release more than one or two mature eggs. A woman undergoing this treatment can go to the clinic for each hormone injection, or she can give the injections to herself, or she can ask someone else, such as her partner or a friend, to give them to her. Most
brands of the injectable hormone are available in "pens" with a
short, fine needle. After some initial help from a nurse, most
women find it quick and painless to administer their own injections. Common side effects of the hormone include headache,
bloating, weight gain, and mood swings. Most women feel minimal side effects, while a few are miserable. Women who experience some or all of these side effects can continue the hormone
treatment as long as they don't have ovarian hyperstimulation syndrome. All side effects go away if pregnancy is not achieved and
menstruation begins.

During a hormone stimulation cycle, the doctor follows the
progress and growth of the eggs with blood tests to check estradiol and luteinizing hormone (LH) levels and with pelvic ultra-

sounds. The ultrasounds are usually done transvaginally, in which a long probe, smaller than a speculum, is inserted into the vagina. The procedure should not cause any more discomfort than a Pap smear. Egg growth can also be monitored with ultrasounds of the abdomen, but a transvaginal ultrasound allows a clearer evaluation of the developing eggs. During a hormone stimulation cycle, the ultrasounds and blood tests may be done every few days, until ovulation. The doctor uses the test results to decide the hormone dose for the subsequent few days and to minimize the risks of overstimulating the ovaries.

With both Clomid and hormone stimulation cycles, some doctors prescribe another hormone, progesterone, to be taken after ovulation. Progesterone can be administered as a pill, a suppository, or a shot. Progesterone is essential to maintain a pregnancy, so there must be adequate levels in the body in case an egg becomes fertilized and implants in the uterus.

INTRAUTERINE INSEMINATION

An additional procedure that can be used with either a Clomid cycle or a hormone stimulation cycle is intrauterine insemination (IUI). In an IUI, the sperm is injected directly into the woman's uterus. The doctor evaluates the woman's blood test and ultrasound results to decide which day during the cycle to perform the IUI. On the day of the IUI, the sperm must be collected in a specimen cup, either at the fertility clinic or at home—provided the sperm can be taken to the clinic's laboratory quickly (generally within 30 to 60 minutes).

Because the sperm will not be going through cervical mucus but will be inserted directly into the uterus, the sperm need to be "washed" in the laboratory to remove substances called prostaglandins. (If unwashed sperm are inserted directly into the uterus, prostaglandins cause the uterus to contract, with severe cramping and, occasionally, a severe allergic reaction. This problem is not encountered with intracervical insemination—ICI, see chapter 4—or with intercourse.) After the sperm have been washed, the doctor or a fertility-trained nurse places them directly into the uterus through a thin tube called a catheter. The procedure should not cause any discomfort and takes only a few minutes. Most doctors recommend that the woman remain lying down for about 10 to 30 minutes following the procedure. She can then resume normal activities.

THE CHANCES OF SUCCESS

Women younger than thirty-five years who undergo hormone stimulation alone or hormone stimulation plus intrauterine insemination have a chance for conception ranging between 5 and 20 percent per cycle. Older women have a lower chance and may be advised to move to more aggressive fertility treatment after only a few cycles, rather than spending a long time trying the early assistance methods.

We hope that you will successfully conceive with early fertility assistance. You and your doctor can discuss how many cycles you wish to try before moving on to more aggressive fertility assistance, called assisted reproductive technology (ART). ART options are described in the next chapter.

FURTHER READING

J. Meyers-Thompson and S. Perkins. *Fertility for Dummies.* Wiley, 2003.

I AM A FORTY-SEVEN-YEAR-OLD married professional. My husband and I got married when I was forty, and we started trying to get pregnant right away. We tried unsuccessfully for six months and then started intrauterine inseminations. After three cycles, I had a laparoscopy, which revealed that both of my tubes were blocked due to endometriosis. So we embarked on IVF (in vitro fertilization). After three unsuccessful attempts, we finally got pregnant with our first son. My husband was happy to stop there, but I had always wanted several children, so he agreed to try again. We tried two more IVF cycles with no success and I was beginning to come to terms with not having more children. I talked my husband into trying one last time, and with this attempt, we became pregnant with twins (a girl and a boy).

The experience was very expensive, because I had no insurance and my age meant I had to take large doses of the fertility medication, resulting in about $10,000 per attempt. It was also time-consuming. I had to take many days off from work for monitoring, egg retrieval, and embryo transfer. The odds were against us with every attempt, having about an 8 to 12 percent chance of success, given my age. The stress was high; I had mood swings from the hormones, both my husband and I worried about our finances, and the process made intimacy a mechanical thing. But looking back, I'd do it all over again. The joys of parenting cannot be described.

Older parents should be aware of a few things, though. While you are probably more patient and financially able when you're older, you should consider the amount of energy that is required and the effect of lack of sleep on your health. We also found that the clinic didn't offer much psychological support, so we recommend that you have a good support system in place before you embark on this process. The clinic did provide a list of counselors to help us address the psychological stresses. Also, the whole process is very mysterious, and I don't think you ever really know what will happen. We were extremely lucky. Being open to options will definitely improve your chances of having the family you want.

———————————————————————————————— ●

Chapter 3

ASSISTED REPRODUCTIVE TECHNOLOGY (ART) USING YOUR OWN EGGS OR SPERM

If you have not conceived with the help of Clomid or hormone stimulation, or if your doctor recommends more aggressive fertility assistance because of your age, the next available option that uses your and your partner's own eggs and sperm is assisted reproductive technology (ART). ART procedures involve laboratory handling of both the woman's eggs and the man's sperm. The most commonly used ART procedure is in vitro fertilization (IVF). The term "in vitro" literally means "in glass," because fertilization of the egg by the sperm occurs in a dish in the laboratory. IVF is an invasive and expensive procedure, and unfortunately it does not guarantee pregnancy. Nevertheless, many couples who use ART (if the woman is younger than forty years) do eventually achieve pregnancy.

THE IVF PROCEDURE

If you decide to go ahead with an IVF treatment, you will find that life becomes highly scheduled for a few weeks as the woman prepares her body for the procedure. She receives hormone shots, or administers them herself, for 10 to 20 days. The length of time depends on how her ovaries respond to the hormone stimulation. The woman will generally make at least four visits to the fertility clinic for blood tests to check hormone levels and ultrasounds to monitor egg growth (similar to the monitoring during hormone stimulation cycles, described in chapter 2). The doctor monitors the test results closely and decides how to adjust the hormone dose. Information on the required dose and timing of the shots is usually relayed to the woman by an IVF nurse. The nurse stays in close contact, almost daily, to give the instructions and to respond to any questions or concerns the woman has. Timing of the shots is critical, particularly for the last hormone shot before the egg retrieval. Depending on what time the eggs are to be retrieved, the final hormone shot may even be scheduled for the middle of the night.

On the day of the egg retrieval, the woman checks in at the clinic sometime in the morning and the man must provide his sperm sample. The woman receives an anesthetic to go lightly to sleep, so that she continues to breathe on her own but is unaware of the surgery being performed. The doctor inserts a probe with a small needle into the vagina and through the vaginal wall and then gently pulls the mature eggs out of the ovaries. The procedure takes 15 to 30 minutes. After the woman wakes up she is watched for a few hours and can then go home. Most women feel fine after the egg retrieval and can go back to work the next day. As with all surgical procedures, there are some medical risks with the egg retrieval for IVF; these risks are discussed in chapter 11.

The eggs and sperm are mixed together in a dish in the fertility center laboratory and, if all goes well, one or more of the eggs will be fertilized. Once an egg is fertilized, it becomes an embryo. The laboratory evaluates and "grades" the embryos according to how robust they are and how well they seem to be growing. Some centers wait until the embryos are at the blastocyst stage, or after about five days of growth, when they have 60 to 100 cells. Waiting for the blastocyst stage can give the doctor a better idea of how well the embryos are developing and can help the decision about which ones to transfer. Transferring only one or two high-quality embryos helps avoid a multiple pregnancy. However, not all embryos will develop to the blastocyst stage. Also, if a couple wants to freeze extra embryos for future IVF attempts, it is preferable to freeze them at earlier stages because these early embryos tolerate the freezing procedure better than blastocysts. Embryo storage is discussed in more detail later in this chapter.

Before you embark on an IVF attempt, you need to think carefully about how many embryos to transfer when the time comes. The fertility specialist discusses this issue with you, and at most centers you will sign documents before beginning the procedure to indicate the number of embryos to transfer and what to do with extra embryos. Transferring several embryos may give a better chance of becoming pregnant, but it increases the risk of having twins, triplets, or even higher-order multiples. The decision also depends on the quality of the embryos, the woman's age, both partners' feelings about fetal termination (discussed in later chapters), and whether or not the fertility center is able to freeze unused embryos. Embryos from older women, particularly those over thirty-five years, have less chance of resulting in a viable pregnancy, so doctors are often willing to transfer more embryos to the uterus of an older woman than for a younger woman.

Transferring the embryos into the woman's uterus is a minor procedure that does not require anesthesia. The doctor slides a thin tube through the cervix and into the uterus, with or without ultrasound guidance, and then slowly inserts the embryos. Some centers recommend bed rest for up to two days after the embryo transfer, whereas other centers do not think bed rest is needed. The woman is also advised to restrict her activities—no heavy lifting, no strenuous exercise, and no intercourse—for a week or two after the transfer. Approximately two weeks after the transfer, the woman has a blood test to determine if she is pregnant.

OVERCOMING MALE FACTOR INFERTILITY

Difficulty conceiving is sometimes caused by a male factor, such as having too few sperm or having abnormal sperm (for example, sperm that do not swim well). If there is any question of a male factor influencing a couple's fertility, another procedure, intracytoplasmic sperm injection (ICSI), can be done in conjunction with

IVF. For ICSI, a single sperm cell—one that has good shape and swims fast—is selected from the sperm sample and injected into the egg. IVF success rates as measured by live births are generally higher when ICSI is used than in cycles where the eggs and sperm are simply mixed together in a dish.

The ICSI procedure can also be combined with microsurgical procedures in which sperm are retrieved directly from the man's testicles—called percutaneous epididymal sperm aspiration (PESA) or testicular sperm extraction (TESE). These procedures can be used in men who have had a vasectomy or have a condition that results in the absence of sperm in the ejaculate.

WHAT DO YOU DO WITH EXTRA EMBRYOS?

Some couples are fortunate enough to make several embryos, more than they want to transfer to the woman's uterus. The fertility center usually gives couples the option of freezing the extra embryos (at additional cost) for future attempts at pregnancy, or donating them for others who need both donor eggs and sperm, or disposing of them in a medically acceptable and ethical manner. Fertility centers counsel patients undergoing IVF on these options and require paperwork to document the option chosen before the IVF procedure begins.

We don't know how long embryos can be frozen and remain viable (meaning, able to progress to a live birth). In the scientific literature, 12 years is reported as the longest period that a human embryo has been stored and then resulted in a live birth after transfer. Deciding to store embryos raises other issues, such as what to do with the embryos in the event of a couple's relationship ending or the death of one partner. These considerations are discussed in chapter 17.

SAVING EGGS FOR FUTURE USE

Can women save their eggs for future use if they are not ready to have children during their "child-bearing" years? Saving eggs may be possible in the future. Eggs can be frozen by using a new technique called vitrification, which is an ultrarapid cooling technique that differs from freezing or conventional cryopreservation. Scientists are currently investigating the use of vitrification and, to date, have mainly used the technique on eggs and embryos, although it is also possible to use it with ovarian tissue. The survival rate for unfertilized eggs has been very good in research settings. Although pregnancies and live births have been achieved with previously frozen eggs, the number of cases is small, so the technique is still considered experimental. We don't yet know the success rate of pregnancy from frozen eggs.

THE CHANCES OF SUCCESS

Assisted reproductive technology methods improve pregnancy rates for women and couples classified as infertile, but the number of successful pregnancies is lower among women over thirty-five years of age than among younger women. The Society for Assisted Reproductive Technology (SART)* released statistics in 2004, summarized in table 3.1, that show the effect of maternal age on the chance of becoming pregnant through IVF treatment using a woman's own eggs. Among women younger than thirty-five years, a successful pregnancy resulted from 1 of every 2.4 cycles attempted (or 10 of every 24 cycles). In contrast, a forty-one-year-old woman had to go through an average of 5 to 6 cycles to become pregnant. The chances of a live birth also declined with maternal age; more than 35 percent of attempted cycles produced a live birth for a woman younger than thirty-five, whereas only about 11 percent did so for a woman aged forty-one or forty-two.

According to the SART data, the chances of a live birth from

---

* SART is an organization affiliated with the American Society for Reproductive Medicine (ASRM). SART's members are the approximately four hundred ART clinics in the United States that submit information every year for SART publications. SART's member clinics are only a proportion of the total number of clinics offering fertility services in the United States, but they most likely give a good overall representation of the statistics on infertile couples and their chances of success with ART procedures.

Table 3.1. Effect of Maternal Age on Cycle Cancellations, Pregnancies, and Live Births for Women Using Their Own Eggs in Assisted Reproductive Technology

Maternal age in years	Cycles canceled	Cycles resulting in pregnancies	Cycles resulting in live births
<35	1/11.9	1/2.4	1/2.7
	(8.4%)	(42.5%)	(36.9%)
35–37	1/8.3	1/2.8	1/3.4
	(12.0%)	(35.5%)	(29.3%)
38–40	1/6.3	1/3.8	1/5.1
	(15.8%)	(26.5%)	(19.5%)
41–42	1/5.1	1/5.8	1/9.3
	(19.5%)	(17.3%)	(10.7%)

Source: Society for Assisted Reproductive Technology data. Centers for Disease Control and Prevention. 2004 Assisted Reproductive Technology (ART) Report: National Summary (http://apps.nccd.cdc.gov/ART2004/nation04.asp).

an attempted cycle plummet as women get even older: 5 percent at age forty-three, and less than 1 percent at age forty-five. Success rates for frozen embryo transfers are slightly lower than those for fresh embryo transfers, because some embryos don't survive the thawing process. The live birth rate per cycle using thawed embryos is 30.6 percent (1 in 3.3) for women younger than thirty-five years. When ICSI is used in an ART cycle, the success rates increase slightly in each maternal age category.

As reported by SART, the proportion of ART cycles that were started and then canceled, usually because there was no or inadequate egg production, increased with maternal age (see table 3.1). Fewer than 10 percent of attempted cycles were canceled for women younger than thirty-five, and nearly 20 percent were canceled for women aged forty-one to forty-two.

Most pregnancies achieved with ART assistance have a good outcome. Pregnancy outcomes of ART cycles from the SART 2004 data are shown in figure 3.1. In total, 81 percent of pregnancies achieved from ART cycles, regardless of a woman's age, resulted in live births.

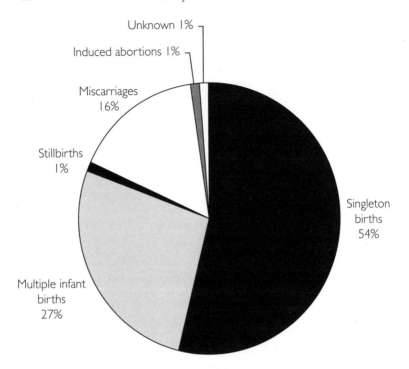

Figure 3.1. Outcomes of pregnancies resulting from assisted reproductive technology (ART) cycles using fresh, nondonor eggs or embryos, 2004. *Source:* Society for Assisted Reproductive Technology data. Centers for Disease Control and Prevention. 2004 Assisted Reproductive Technology (ART) Report: National Summary (http://apps.nccd.cdc.gov/ART2004/nation04.asp).

NEXT STEPS

Fertility assistance cannot guarantee anyone a baby. What should you do if you have gone through some or all of the fertility assisted options, including IVF, and still have not conceived using your own eggs and sperm? You can try IVF again (and again), or you can think about moving on to another option. Your doctor may recommend a certain pathway, such as using donor eggs, donor embryos, or surrogacy, depending on your situation. The following chapters describe what to expect if you decide to pursue any of these pathways.

FURTHER READING

S. L. Cooper and E. S. Glazer. *Choosing Assisted Reproduction: Social, Emotional, Ethical Considerations.* Perspectives Press, 1998.
J. Meyers-Thompson and S. Perkins. *Fertility for Dummies.* Wiley, 2003.

I HAD AN UNPLANNED PREGNANCY when I was seventeen, and I willingly gave the baby up for adoption. I knew I wouldn't be able to look after a baby, especially with the baby's father gone from my life. I married at the age of twenty-nine, and my husband and I started trying to get pregnant. Because of my teen pregnancy, I had always thought that I'd have no trouble getting pregnant again. I was wrong. Nothing happened after months of trying. My husband and I were both checked out by a fertility doctor, and it turned out that my husband had a low sperm count and very few of the sperm he did have were motile. This news came as a huge shock to my husband, who is a big, tall, very masculine guy. The doctor told us that if we wanted to have our own biological children, we should really consider in vitro fertilization with a special technique where a single sperm is injected into each of my eggs. The technique is called intracytoplasmic sperm injection, and neither of us had ever heard of it, but we were willing to give it a try. We really, really wanted to have children with our own eggs and sperm.

I began the hormone stimulation to mature my eggs, and when they were big enough I had the egg retrieval procedure. My husband gave a sperm sample, and then the lab people got to work. They created four embryos, but only one developed well enough to transfer. Two weeks after this embryo was placed into my uterus, I was to go for a blood test to check for the pregnancy hormone. I began to bleed that morning, and the test confirmed that I wasn't pregnant. We went through the IVF and ICSI procedure three more times. On the second and third times, I didn't become pregnant, despite having two good embryos to transfer each time. On the fourth attempt, I did get pregnant, and this time with twins. Finally! We were so excited, especially at the thought of having an instant family.

At 11 weeks into the pregnancy I began to bleed and I was terrified. I phoned my doctor, who told me to go right to the hospital to find out what was going on. I miscarried one of the babies, but the other stayed put and continued to develop. I was sad at losing the baby and also relieved and grateful to still be pregnant. Our son was born three weeks before his due date and is doing just great.

Chapter 4

USING DONOR SPERM

The decision to use donor sperm is usually an early one. You may be a single woman or a lesbian couple trying for a pregnancy, or you may be a heterosexual couple whose fertility workup identified a problem with the man's sperm. About 50,000 children are born each year in the United States as a result of donor sperm insemination.

Insemination with donor sperm causes minimal interruption to a woman's daily schedule. Most often, two or three inseminations are done around the time when the woman ovulates during her monthly cycle. Women with a 28-day cycle usually ovulate on day 14. Women with shorter or longer cycles can use basal body temperature monitoring to identify when they ovulate. The sperm must be present in the uterus just before or within about 12 hours of ovulation for the greatest chance of an egg being fertilized.

The insemination procedure is relatively easy: a doctor or nurse at the fertility clinic inserts the sperm sample either just inside the cervical opening (intracervical insemination, or ICI) or directly into the uterus (intrauterine insemination, or IUI). ICIs are less expensive than IUIs because, with an ICI, the sperm must make their own way through the cervical mucus and so they don't need to be washed first. For an IUI, the sperm must be washed to remove prostaglandins (substances that cause the uterus to contract) before they are released into the uterus. Both insemination procedures are done with a thin, flexible catheter, and neither procedure should cause more discomfort than a regular Pap smear. The woman is usually encouraged to rest for about 10 to 30 minutes after the sperm have been inserted, but she can otherwise resume normal activities. Although slightly more costly, IUIs have a higher success rate than ICIs.

The donor sperm can be obtained from a fertility clinic, a sperm donor bank, or a known donor. Regardless of the source, the sperm must always be screened for sexually transmitted diseases. With unscreened sperm the woman is at risk of contracting a serious infection, including human immunodeficiency virus (HIV). Donor sperm samples are also routinely screened for certain genetic disorders.

ANONYMOUS DONORS

If you decide to use donor sperm from a fertility center or a sperm bank, you will have a lot of choices. In addition to being carefully screened for both genetic and infectious diseases, sperm donors generally must meet other requirements, too:

- Height: Most requests are for donors between 5 feet 10 inches and 6 feet 2 inches.
- Weight: The donor's weight should be proportional to his height.
- Age: The donor should be between the ages of nineteen and thirty-nine.
- Education: The donor may be a graduate of a four-year college program, and at the least he will have completed two years of college.
- Sperm: The donor's sample must have a high sperm count (at least 20 million/ml is considered a normal count), 70 percent of the sperm must be motile (moving), and 60 percent must have a normal appearance.

The donor profile also includes data such as ethnic origin, description of personality, likes and dislikes, family history, and so forth. Donor profiles can be extensive and may include a section in which the donor has been asked to write his motivation for donation and a personal message. To get an idea of how extensive the choices are, search for sperm donors on the internet and review sample donor profiles.

Guidelines of the American Society for Reproductive Medicine suggest that a donor be allowed to father no more than 10 children. Sperm banks routinely follow up with questionnaires to fertility centers that use donor sperm to find out if a donation resulted in a live birth.

When men donate their sperm, they sign documents to give up their parental rights and to be protected from parental responsibilities. Some sperm banks now have donors who have agreed to be contacted when the child is eighteen years old. The child can get in touch with the donor directly, or the clinic can notify the donor on the child's request. Mothers who belong to a national organization called Single Mothers by Choice are setting up a sibling registry, so that children who are biologically connected by the same donor will be able to contact one another.

KNOWN (DIRECTED) DONORS

Some people prefer to have more information about the sperm donor or to use a donor who is related to the woman's partner. Regardless of whether a known donor is a friend or a relative, the donor and sperm must be screened for infectious diseases. Sperm banks freeze their sperm samples, but if you know the donor, fresh sperm can be used for the insemination. The pregnancy rate is higher when fresh sperm are used.

THE CHANCES OF SUCCESS

The chances of a woman becoming pregnant with donor sperm range from 5 to 19 percent and are similar to the chances of conception among the general population, provided the woman doesn't have fertility problems herself. On average, in the general population, women younger than thirty have about a 20 percent chance of conceiving in any given cycle; this rate decreases with maternal age to about 15 percent at ages thirty to thirty-five and less than 10 percent over age thirty-five.

FURTHER READING

T. M. Erickson and M. Lathus. *Assisted Reproduction: The Complete Guide to Having a Baby with the Help of a Third Party.* iUniverse, 2005.
C. F. Vercollone, H. Moss, and R. Moss. *Helping the Stork: The Choices and Challenges of Donor Insemination.* Macmillan, 1997.

BECAUSE MY HUSBAND IS TRANSGENDERED, we knew that the only way I could get pregnant was through artificial insemination. We briefly considered using a friend as a donor, but decided that being so close to the biological father might be emotionally awkward for him, for us, and someday for our child. So we opted to use an anonymous donor.

Our fertility specialist worked with several cryobanks. They all had donor databases online, so we could search profiles from home. Cryobanks offer free basic information on all their donors, such as height, hair and eye color, weight, age, and level of education. However, we had to pay extra fees to view a photo of a donor as an infant or to find out about the medical history of a donor and his family.

At first I thought, "How are we going to pick someone?" It seemed a daunting task and somewhat odd, as if we were ordering a child from a menu. However, once my husband said we should pick someone with his characteristics, I gained focus and became more comfortable. We tried to find someone who not only looked like my husband (dark hair, brown eyes, Caucasian, etc.), but also had similar interests and a similar personality.

To give a sense of donors' personalities, cryobank questionnaires cover things like favorite color, favorite food, artistic abilities, interests in travel, and life goals. Donors are also asked to describe their personality. The donor we selected seemed a lot like my husband and said he had an outgoing personality and a good sense of humor. Of course, we had to trust that donors answer honestly.

Fortunately, some cryobanks also provide staff impressions of donors, including comments about donors' personality and appearance. Our donor was described as friendly and outgoing with a boyish face. Because donors are anonymous, cryobanks don't provide photos of them as adults. So staff impressions can mean a lot. One cryobank even described facial features, such as chin strength, cheek bone height, nose size, and eye setting.

Although I became comfortable searching databases for donors, I continued to have mixed feelings about being inseminated with a stranger's sperm. On a primal level, carrying a stranger's child seemed unnatural. But I realized I was being much more sentimental about this transaction than the donor, who indicated in the questionnaire that he was donating sperm to help people have children and to pay his college tuition.

I did have other concerns about using an anonymous donor. I realized that if someday my child needed a transplant and I weren't a match, I wouldn't be able to turn to his biological father or half siblings. I rationalized that parents and siblings aren't always a match anyway and we would have to take this chance.

I was even more concerned about telling our child how he was conceived. I wondered when the best time would be and if he would be upset about never being able to meet his biological father. Fortunately, our fertility specialist required all of his patients to meet with a psychologist. She recommended that we create a photo album, telling the story of how our child came to be. She said the first page should have a photo or magazine cutout of a doctor holding a package. Initially, we could tell our child that we had to wait for a special package to arrive and the doctor used it to help me get pregnant. She said that as our child gets older and asks more questions, we could add more age-appropriate details. She stressed that keeping the artificial insemination a secret until our child was a teenager would not be healthy for him. Essentially, she said, he should always know his conception was special so he won't be shocked when he hears all the details.

After selecting the donor, who was identified by number, we phoned in the order. Of course, we had hoped I would get pregnant the next time I ovulated, but I didn't. Some of my hormone levels were off, and my doctor couldn't attempt insemination again until they reached normal levels. I had to change my diet and take a fertility drug to fix that problem. It took three months for my hormones to reach levels at which pregnancy was possible. Two months later, the second attempt at insemination worked.

When the nurse told me I was pregnant, I was ecstatic and no longer cared that I would never meet the donor. To me, #3709 is just a number. My husband is my son's father in every way that matters. Yes, telling our son that he was conceived using donor sperm and that his father is transgendered will be difficult, but I hope the love and support we give him will enable him to take both these facts in stride.

Chapter 5

USING DONOR EGGS
AND EMBRYOS

Most couples go through all or most other fertility assistance options using their own eggs and sperm before they choose to try donor eggs or embryos. Using donor eggs or embryos is more complicated than using donor sperm. To donate eggs or embryos, the donor must go through an in vitro fertilization (IVF) procedure, as described in chapter 3. Also, the donor and the recipient must synchronize their menstrual cycles so that the recipient's body is ready to receive the implanted embryo or embryos when they are at the optimal stage of development. Despite the additional complications, egg donation is a growing national trend, and an increasing number of fertility clinics now offer donor egg and donor embryo services as one of their fertility assistance options. In 2004, more than 13,000 cycles used donor eggs or embryos, and at the time of writing this book, approximately 30,000 babies had been born in the United States as a result of egg or embryo donation.

Once an egg or embryo donor has been identified, the woman who will receive the embryo—the recipient—must synchronize her menstrual cycle with the donor's cycle to prepare her uterus for embryo implantation. The synchronization usually begins the month before the transfer, and the recipient typically has a schedule of both injections and pills. The embryo transfer is done in the same way as described for IVF (see chapter 3), and the recipient is usually prescribed another hormone, progesterone, to support the pregnancy after the transfer. A woman who lives in a different state from the egg donor will need to travel to the fertility center in the donor's state for the embryo transfer, but the preparatory hormone therapy and all follow-up care can generally be done in the recipient's home state. Depending on logistics and local state regulations, the transfer of a donated embryo can be performed either at the clinic where the embryo was created and stored or at a clinic where the recipient lives. However, it is safest not to move embryos and to do the transfer where the embryos are stored. Women who have already been through an IVF cycle tend to find that being an egg or embryo recipient is much easier in several respects, since it is the donor who undergoes the intense hormone stimulation to produce multiple mature eggs.

Psychological screening is a standard practice for recipients of donor eggs and embryos. The purpose of the screening is to assess the woman's psychological readiness to carry a fetus that is not genetically related to her and to review long-term issues that will come up, such as how or if the woman intends to disclose the method of conception to her child.

DONOR EGGS

Donor eggs may be available either from a fertility center that offers egg donation as one of its services or through a donor agency with the sole purpose of identifying donors. Donor agencies collaborate with medical programs to make matches between their donors and potential recipients.

Donor eggs can't be screened in a comparable way to donor sperm, which can be assessed for quality—appearance and movement. Therefore, it isn't possible to know the quality of a donor egg before it is used, and there are no guarantees that the egg will not carry a genetic abnormality. Nevertheless, egg donors must meet certain criteria that should minimize the chances for age-related or other effects on the eggs they donate. Egg donors must usually be younger than thirty-five years of age, be in good health, and have no history of inheritable diseases.

Anonymous Egg Donors

How do fertility centers and donor agencies find their egg donors? They usually draw from the general population by advertising through the media, such as in local papers, magazines, or university publications. The internet has also become a popular tool to find donors. Another source is women who have chosen to have their fallopian tubes tied (tubal ligation) to prevent further pregnancies. These women may be offered a free or reduced rate for the ligation procedure in return for donating eggs.

Donor agencies are set up to accept applications from possible donors (as well as from recipients). Not all applicants are accepted as donors. Women interested in donating eggs generally must go through a rigorous screening process, which includes an extensive family history, blood tests to check for inheritable diseases, and psychological assessment. Donors who are in a high-risk group for specific disorders may undergo additional screening for these diseases. Ideally, donors are women who have chosen to donate their eggs primarily for philanthropic reasons. If you decide to pursue becoming a recipient of donor eggs, you can review the selection process that was used to find the eggs.

When using donor eggs through a fertility center, the recipients probably won't have a panel of donors to choose from, as they would with donor sperm. Egg recipients are usually placed on a waiting list, and when a donor becomes available they are given the option to use her eggs. The recipients receive only basic information about the egg donor, such as her age, what she looks like (phenotypic characteristics), her family history of diseases, and her education and interests. Anonymous donors at fertility centers routinely receive compensation from the recipients, and the amount differs by center. Some centers also offer the opportunity to share donor eggs with another recipient or to match a recipient with a fellow infertility patient who agrees to share her eggs if the recipient pays her IVF costs. These strategies can decrease the total cost, but recipients have less freedom in their choices and possibly fewer good eggs for transfer.

Some centers work with donor agencies or have a registry of donors where recipients can search for specific characteristics. For example, if everyone in a woman's family has red hair and she wants a red-haired donor, she can probably find one. A search of "egg donation programs" on the internet yields thousands of responses, which are mainly for donor agencies and fertility centers with egg donation programs, many with donor egg registries. By going through a donor agency, recipients have more choice of donor eggs and can usually obtain a lot of information about each donor before making a selection.

Many agencies also have donor egg programs that are called "exceptional" or "extraordinary." Donors who qualify for these programs must meet specific criteria with their educational achievements. Using such a donor does not guarantee that the child will be a genius, but the eggs—and therefore the genetic material—have come from an individual who has achieved success, probably through a combination of intelligence and hard work. Of course, eggs from exceptional or extraordinary donors are more expensive, since these donors often request higher compensation.

A child born from a donor egg is automatically the child of the recipients and does not need to be legally adopted by either parent at birth. Donors must sign documents stating that they are voluntarily donating their eggs and will not claim any parenting rights in the future. It's advisable to get legal counsel when going through the process of using donor eggs (see chapter 17).

Known (Directed) Egg Donors

Some people who use donor eggs want a genetic link to the donor or want to know who the donor is. Sometimes recipients meet the egg donor solely for the purpose of the egg donation, but most known donors are family members (sisters, cousins, nieces, and possibly daughters) or friends. Using a family member or friend will generally be less expensive, since the donor isn't usually financially compensated, although her medical costs for the IVF treatment must still be covered by the recipient. Known donors must also be screened for infectious and genetic diseases.

DONOR EMBRYOS

Using a donor embryo, also termed "embryo adoption," is an option for single women who can't use their own eggs or for couples who can contribute neither eggs nor sperm to the process. A woman or a couple can follow one of two pathways when they decide to use a donor embryo. They can have a preexisting embryo donated by the genetic parents or they can intentionally create an embryo through egg and sperm donations. Although using either of these pathways creates an embryo that is not genetically connected to the parent or parents, several differences exist between the two. Creating an embryo allows more control, but it also increases the emotional, financial, and hassle costs.

Preexisting embryo donation occurs relatively infrequently. As of winter 1997, only about 150 babies in the United States had been born from donated, rather than created, embryos, possibly because of the shortage of available embryos for donation. Most couples who undergo IVF with their own eggs and sperm eventually transfer (that is, use) all their embryos, and those who don't often feel uncomfortable donating their embryos. Recently, a private fertility center in Texas (The Abraham Center of Life) has been making embryos for unspecified recipients, and it then matches embryos to client preferences.

Preexisting frozen (cryopreserved) embryos and donor gametes (donor eggs and sperm) that can be used to create embryos are available through most fertility clinics for couples who can't use their own eggs and sperm. There are also brokers who use the internet or organizations dedicated to egg and embryo donation to match embryos that couples are willing to donate with prospective parents. The recipients of an embryo receive information about the donating parents and usually a family genetic history. Using a donor embryo is considered to be an adoption, albeit at the embryo level, so if you decide to take this pathway you may have to undergo a home study (home studies are described in chapter 15).

Like sperm and egg donation, preexisting embryo donation can be anonymous or known (directed). In an anonymous donation of a preexisting embryo, the fertility clinic usually selects the embryo recipient. The clinic tries to match the donor and recipient in terms of their ethnicity and what they look like (phenotypic characteristics). Recipients are given information about the donors so that they can decide if they want to accept the embryo or embryos. In a known or directed donation, the donor couple has input into selecting the embryo recipient. The donor couple may also request to know if a pregnancy occurs and even to have ongoing contact with the recipient after the baby's birth, although the couple has no parental rights or responsibilities.

EGG RECONSTITUTION TECHNIQUES

The greatest concern that many women have about using donor eggs is the loss of a genetic link. For this reason, researchers are looking at methods to reconstitute eggs that are impaired because of a woman's age or for other reasons. Developments in reproductive technology now make it possible to reconstruct eggs and embryos from the various components of an egg (nucleus, cytoplasm, cytoplasmic organelles). The components can be gathered from several different eggs. This procedure is still being researched and isn't yet available—but it's a technology to look for in the future.

Another procedure, already available at some fertility centers, is cytoplasmic transfer. Cytoplasmic transfer is an assisted reproductive technology (ART) procedure that takes a small amount of cytoplasm (the viscous semifluid inside an egg) from a donor egg and injects it into the recipient's own egg with the goal of enhancing the quality of the embryo. Very little or no genetic material (DNA) is transferred from the donor egg, so the recipient maintains her genetic link to the egg. Cytoplasmic transfer may be recommended for women with a history of poor embryo quality to increase the likelihood that the embryos will develop. The procedure is generally not done in women over the age of forty because of the higher probability of a genetic abnormality, and, as mentioned, cytoplasmic transfer does not alter the genetic makeup of the egg.

When a woman undergoes cytoplasmic transfer, the procedure is combined with intracytoplasmic sperm injection (ICSI), in which a sperm cell is injected into the egg (as described in chapter 3). So both the sperm and the donor cytoplasm are injected into the egg at the same time. Currently, cytoplasmic transfer is only done using the cytoplasm of fresh donor eggs, but studies are underway using cytoplasm from frozen donor eggs. A 1998 survey of fertility centers noted that fewer than 5 percent offered cytoplasmic transfer, but more may have this service available in the future.

THE CHANCES OF SUCCESS

The chance of pregnancy and live birth with donor eggs depends primarily on the donor's age, not the recipient's. Because egg donors are usually required to be younger than thirty-five years, the success rates are quite high. According to statistics from the Society for Assisted Reproductive Technology, half (50.2%) of cycles that used donor eggs resulted in a live birth. Although there are no data for donor embryos specifically, frozen embryo transfers overall resulted in pregnancy in about one-third (31.7%) of attempts for women younger than thirty-five years.

FURTHER READING

Centers for Disease Control and Prevention. Assisted Reproductive Technology (ART) Report. 2004. Available at: www.cdc.gov/ART/ART2004.

S. L. Cooper and E. S. Glazer. *Choosing Assisted Reproduction: Social, Emotional, Ethical Considerations.* Perspectives Press, 1998.

T. M. Erickson and M. Lathus. *Assisted Reproduction: The Complete Guide to Having a Baby with the Help of a Third Party.* iUniverse, 2005.

E. S. Glazer and E. W. Sterling. *Having Your Baby through Egg Donation.* Perspectives Press, 2003.

J. Meyers-Thompson and S. Perkins. *Fertility for Dummies.* Wiley, 2003.

C. F. Vercollone, H. Moss, and R. Moss. *Helping the Stork: The Choices and Challenges of Donor Insemination.* Macmillan, 1997.

● ───

I ALWAYS THOUGHT I'D HAVE CHILDREN in the future, but I was so caught up in work and life that I didn't get serious about becoming a parent until my mid-thirties. My partner and I weren't married, but we were in a long-term relationship and we decided we were ready for children. After trying to conceive for a few years, we sought fertility assistance (which was not covered by my insurance). When I was thirty-nine we began trying IVF, but were not successful after three attempts. At that point, we contemplated international adoption versus donor eggs. A domestic adoption was less appealing because we didn't want to sell ourselves to a birth mother for an independent adoption, and we didn't want to have a possible wait of several years for an agency adoption. Any adoption would have been difficult because we still weren't married. My partner also really wanted a genetic link, and I was nervous about the potential long-term effects that the early environment has on international adoptees. So we opted for donor eggs.

Our state did not have any donor egg programs, so we chose a program in the city of my birth. This appealed to us because we could stay with family and the source pool was genetically my background. We had to wait a few months for an evaluation at the fertility center, and then we were put on a waiting list. About a year later, we received a call that we were next on the list. When a donor became available we received a fax with limited information, including the donor's appearance, her likes and dislikes, her education, and her family history. We then had to respond quickly if we wanted to use this egg donor. The first donor backed out, but the second donor agreed. Fortunately, from what I could tell, her physical appearance was similar to mine, and she had a genetic background very like mine.

We flew into town a few days before the egg retrieval. The eggs were inseminated with my partner's sperm and several embryos were viable. The transfer was very easy and took about 30 minutes. We flew back home and were ecstatic two weeks later when my pregnancy test was positive. Apart from a threatened miscarriage at around 7 or 8 weeks, for which I went on bed rest for a week, our pregnancy was uneventful.

When I was forty-two years old, I gave birth to healthy twins, a boy and a girl, at nearly 39 weeks gestation. Our children resemble their father greatly and look enough like me that nobody thinks to ask questions. Last year when they turned six years old, I explained to both children that they were from donor eggs. My daughter was very attentive and asked extremely specific questions about the process, but I think the whole conversation went over my son's head. When she's mad at me, my daughter sometimes yells that I am not her real mother, and my son has told me I am not part of the family. I was prepared for these kinds of outburst, but I wasn't really ready for my daughter to start sobbing on a few occasions that she wants to meet her egg mother. I also wasn't prepared to have my daughter call me her "non-egg" mother in public. Regardless of these situations, I am still more comfortable with not keeping our children's origins a secret.

In retrospect, I would have done everything the same way—except I would have turned to donor eggs after only one or two IVF attempts, knowing that our chance for conception with my eggs was very low. Our children are the center of our lives and I cannot now imagine life without them.

Chapter 6

USING A SURROGATE

For one reason or another, some women are unable to carry a pregnancy. For these women, having a surrogate carry the pregnancy for them may be an option. A surrogate can be one of two types, traditional or gestational, and a surrogacy program can be either open or closed. A traditional surrogate is inseminated with the sperm of the intended father or with donor sperm, and the resulting child is genetically related to the surrogate. A gestational surrogate has an embryo placed into her uterus, but the surrogate's egg is not used to create the embryo. In an open program, surrogates and couples are introduced to each other. A surrogate may meet many couples before she selects one, and couples may meet many surrogates before they make their selection. Once they've met and selected each other, the surrogate and the couple interact closely throughout the process of insemination or embryo transfer, pregnancy, and delivery. In a closed program, couples receive biographical information and a photograph, and then they choose their surrogate. The couple and the surrogate meet only once before the child's birth to finalize the stepparent adoption, and once more after the birth for their court appearance, if this is required (see chapter 17).

FINDING A SURROGATE

Surrogacy arrangements may be done independently or through an agency; some agencies only provide assistance for one type of surrogacy (gestational or traditional). Many surrogacy agencies, particularly large ones, will assist with the matching, psychological testing, and legal aspects of using a surrogate. Smaller agencies may only assist with finding a surrogate and then provide referrals for psychological testing and legal counsel. Some fertility centers also offer surrogacy services and can assist with the arrangements.

Surrogacy programs vary in the criteria they require for a woman to be accepted as a surrogate, but all programs have some minimum criteria. The potential surrogate usually must be of a certain age (for example, between twenty-five and thirty-five years), healthy, and, ideally, known to be fertile (by having had at least one child). She must go through the same extensive screening described in the previous chapters for inheritable diseases and sexually transmitted diseases. She must also undergo a psychological assessment to evaluate whether she is emotionally stable and psychologically prepared to be a surrogate. The counselor will explore several questions including some "what if" scenarios such as miscarriage, giving birth to a handicapped child, developing a bond to the unborn child, regretting her decision to relinquish the child, something unanticipated happening to the intended parents, and the child approaching her in years to come.

With both traditional and gestational surrogacy, there are obvious cautions concerning a woman's motivation to be a surrogate. Although surrogate mothers have received criticism that they do it for financial gain (and perhaps some do), most surrogates screened through agencies are women who meet certain criteria, such as having a history of physically and emotionally enjoyable pregnancies, having a close relationship with their own children, living in a supportive home environment, and believing that giving the gift of parenthood would be a positive emotional experience.

Agencies typically ask both parties to write a letter—"Dear Intended Parents" and "Dear Surrogate"—about why they want to be a surrogate and why they are pursuing surrogacy. Chapter 15 provides details of what should be included in the letters. The agency makes matches on the basis of the information in the letters, the results of the psychological screening of both surrogate and intended parents, and the amount of emotional support the intended parents can or cannot provide to the surrogate. The time it takes to match intended parents with a potential surrogate varies; in larger agencies, the average wait is one to three months. When a match is made, both parties must agree to the match before the arrangement can be formalized and proceed.

WORKING WITH A SURROGATE

When a surrogate's pregnancy has been established as viable, the intended parents have many long months to wait as their baby develops. Unfortunately, these months may not be free of anxiety. The intended parents may want genetic testing or an amniocentesis to be performed, and they may also want the right to decide if the pregnancy should be terminated. However, these decisions are exclusively the right of the surrogate, regardless of a legal contract. Most agencies will work with the intended parents and their surrogate to negotiate these procedures, and some surrogates leave these decisions entirely to the intended parents.

The main disadvantage for intended parents in surrogacy arrangements is that they can't dictate the fetal environment, nor can they change their minds if the child is born with defects or special needs, even if the complications were caused by some behavior of the surrogate. If the surrogate is participating in activities that the intended parents believe to be unhealthy for the fetus, there is little they can do unless the agency monitors the situation and intervenes. Some agencies allow drug screening if the intended parents feel this is necessary. In many surrogacy arrangements, however, such problems can be avoided because the intended parents and surrogate have time to get to know each other and to build a trusting and often very strong relationship.

After a surrogate gives birth, there is generally some contact between the parents and the surrogate for a while, but the contact typically diminishes over time, particularly with gestational surrogates. A traditional surrogate, as the biological mother, may have more and continued contact with the parents if the amount of contact was written into the arrangement.

THE LEGALITY OF SURROGACY

There is no national policy on surrogacy, and laws governing surrogacy arrangements vary from state to state. Legislation on surrogacy is also constantly changing. Many current state laws are the result of cases that have gone to court, where the judge writes the laws with each ruling. Most laws focus on the binding contract and payment for services. In most states, there is no provision for surrogacy in state law, and individual judges may have complete discretion when deciding whether or not to issue birth orders, which allows placement of the name(s) of the intended parent(s) on the original birth certificate, or to enforce an agreement between the intended parents and the surrogate. Laws and practices are also likely to differ depending on whether surrogacy is traditional or gestational.

Some states have implemented programs and legal provisions to assist couples and individuals in building a family through surrogacy, most often for gestational surrogacy arrangements. Legal statutes exist in some states to allow the intended parents' names to go directly on the birth certificate, thus circumventing the need for adoption after the child is born (although certain states, such as Texas, permit this only for married heterosexual couples). Elsewhere, whoever gives birth is the legal mother, regardless of the child's genetic makeup, and the intended parents must go through an adoption procedure.

According to 2004 data from Human Rights Campaign, some states classify surrogacy arrangements as "permitted" (that is, allowing individuals and couples to enter into surrogacy contracts), others classify them as "prohibited" (not allowing individuals and couples to enter into surrogacy contracts in all or some instances), and still others have mixed or unclear state laws and/or court case rulings that make it difficult to determine whether or not surrogacy agreements are allowed. Six states allow individuals and couples to enter into surrogacy contracts: Arkansas, California, Illinois (gestational surrogacy only), Massachusetts, New Jersey (uncompensated surrogacy agreements only), and Washington (uncompensated surrogacy agreements only). In the District of Columbia and 11 states, surrogacy agreements are prohibited in all or some instances. Indiana and Louisiana prohibit traditional surrogacy; Michigan and Nebraska prohibit compensated surrogacy agreements; and the District of Columbia, Florida, Nevada, New York, North Dakota, Texas, Utah, and Virginia prohibit surrogacy for all unmarried couples. The remaining 33 states have mixed or unclear laws on surrogacy.

People who live in a state that lacks a surrogacy-friendly legislature are not prevented from engaging in a legal surrogacy arrangement. The laws regarding a surrogacy arrangement depend on the state in which the birth takes place and how those laws are interpreted. More information on legal considerations is provided in chapter 17.

GESTATIONAL SURROGACY

Gestational surrogates are women who carry a pregnancy with eggs donated from the intended mother or an egg donor and sperm donated from the intended father or a sperm donor. Gestational surrogates make it possible for women without a uterus and women who suffer recurrent miscarriages to have children. Gestational surrogacy (also called IVF—in vitro fertilization—surrogacy) arrangements are usually set up either as independent adoptions (in states where this is legal) or by contracts through an agency. Some women prefer the surrogate to be someone they don't already know, while others feel comfortable with a family member (such as a sister) or a close friend acting as the surrogate. Arrangements with a relative or friend are often made directly through a fertility center, not an agency. Private arrangements generally require legal counsel to ensure that the intended parent or parents are registered on the birth certificate as the legal parents.

In 2004, according to data from the Society for Assisted Reproductive Technology (SART), 76 of 411 U.S. fertility centers offered gestational surrogacy services. Gestational surrogates have delivered an estimated 10,000 babies in the United States since 1976. This number may be an underestimate, though, because private gestational surrogacy arrangements may not be reported, particularly in states where the procedure is illegal.

When a gestational carrier has been found and an agreement put in place, the next step is to create an embryo and implant it in the carrier's uterus. The intended mother or the egg donor (see chapter 5 for information on finding an egg donor) has her eggs harvested for the IVF procedure. It isn't necessary to undergo hormone stimulation to obtain the eggs if the woman ovulates consistently. A woman usually produces one or two eggs in a natural, nonstimulated cycle. The woman is monitored with ultrasounds, and once her eggs have reached a specific size, she receives one hormone shot to assist with ovulation. The eggs are then retrieved by laparoscopy. Natural, nonstimulated cycles are less expensive than stimulated cycles and do not have the risks that accompany hormone stimulation. The retrieved eggs are fertilized with the intended father's sperm or donor sperm in an IVF procedure (see chapter 3) and an embryo is inserted into the surrogate, who has undergone hormone therapy to prepare herself as the embryo recipient. The surrogate must agree not to have sexual intercourse with anyone for a specified period of time both before and after the embryo transfer (typically two weeks pre- and post-transfer). As with traditional IVF treatment, a pregnancy test is usually done two weeks after the embryo transfer.

The intended parents take custody of the child immediately after delivery. They then petition the court for approval of the surrogacy agreement, and the legal adoption process begins. The court examines the agreement and confirms the intended parents as the legal parents, unless there is some problem. In some states, the legal parentage can be arranged at the beginning of the process, before the embryo transfer.

TRADITIONAL SURROGACY

Traditional surrogates are both the biological mother and the pregnancy carrier. In other words, a traditional surrogate uses her own eggs for the pregnancy. The intended father provides the sperm or donor sperm are used, and the surrogate undergoes insemination with either an intrauterine insemination (IUI) or intracervical insemination (ICI) procedure (see chapters 2 and 4) at the fertility center. The man who provides the sperm for insemination (whether intended father or sperm donor) must be screened for infections, as described in chapter 4 for sperm donation.

The obvious risk in traditional surrogacy is that the surrogate, as the biological mother, has complete rights to keep the child, regardless of any contract entered into prior to conception. To avoid this risk, many couples opt to use a gestational surrogate instead.

Traditional surrogacy is a hybrid of surrogacy and adoption. Immediately after the child's birth and confirmation of the child's paternity, the court enters an order affirming the intended father's parental status as the biological and legal father. The surrogate's consent to give up the child is obtained after delivery, and then the intended mother files a petition to adopt the child as a stepparent. In some states, a home study is required and can be completed before the delivery. The court reviews the case and, if it's approved, names the intended parents as the legal parents and orders the issuance of a new birth certificate.

THE CHANCES OF SUCCESS

The chance of pregnancy and a live birth when using a surrogate depends largely on the age and fertility of the surrogate for traditional surrogacy and on the age of the egg donor for gestational surrogacy. In traditional surrogacy, successful pregnancies result at a rate of 5 to 15 percent per cycle (which is similar to the pregnancy rate with artificial insemination). In gestational surrogacy, the chances of a successful pregnancy when the intended mother uses her own eggs are the same as those discussed in chapter 3 (see table 3.1), and when donor eggs are used, the chances are as described in chapter 5.

Although the surrogacy option may seem fraught with complications and uncertainties, it is an option that has worked successfully for many, many people. If it's an option that you think could work for you, do as much background research as you can and seek experts to help you navigate the intricacies of finding a surrogate and setting up a workable arrangement.

FURTHER READING

T. M. Erickson and M. Lathus. *Assisted Reproduction: The Complete Guide to Having a Baby with the Help of a Third Party.* iUniverse, 2005.

Human Rights Campaign. Surrogacy Laws: State by State. 2004. Available at: www.hrc.org.

G. Sutton. *A Matter of Trust: The Guide to Gestational Surrogacy.* Clouds Publishing, 1997.

TASC: The American Surrogacy Center. www.surrogacy.com.

I AM THIRTY-NINE YEARS OLD and have been through seven IVF cycles. I got pregnant with four of the cycles, but I miscarried them all. The furthest I ever got was 14 weeks. I had a tubal problem, with both my fallopian tubes blocked right where they join the uterus, and the doctors thought IVF would be the only treatment I'd need. But, after the fourth miscarriage, an ultrasound showed my uterus to be enlarged with fibroids. My doctor recommended removing the fibroids before another attempt at IVF. During the surgery, they found that my uterus was not enlarged from fibroids but because of a disease called adenomyosis, which is endometrial tissue in the wall of the uterus. It wasn't clear if I could ever carry my own child. If I did get pregnant and reach 20 or more weeks, would my uterus hold up and not rupture?

I was emotionally burned out from the pregnancy losses and then the news about my uterus. My husband didn't want to try again; he couldn't bear the thought of another pregnancy loss. So, I began to think about our other options, which were adoption, surrogacy, and not having children. My husband was vehemently opposed to adoption because he was concerned that he wouldn't bond with a child who wasn't genetically his. I couldn't live with childlessness, so our remaining option was surrogacy. It was a painful emotional journey to think about using a surrogate. I felt so out of control in having to ask someone else to carry our child. I began to see family members and friends as potential carriers. It was driving me insane.

After many counseling sessions with a psychologist and hours discussing it with my husband, we decided to look for a surrogate. I researched centers in several states, and finally settled on one in California. We liked California's progressive laws about surrogacy, and the center's director was warm and supportive. It was easy signing a contract, but selecting a surrogate wasn't so easy. I looked at package after package and video after video trying to select just the right person. I finally chose our surrogate candidate, and we flew out to meet her and decide if the fit was right. She was very nice, but it still felt awkward. I agonized some more about the decision. Finally, we agreed to proceed and our surrogacy contracts were signed.

It was challenging to coordinate the surrogate's and my menstrual cycles and to estimate when my egg retrieval would occur. My husband and I are busy professionals so it was hard to set aside a week when both of us could fly across the country for our IVF cycle. We finally got everything scheduled and had the procedure. We flew back home and waited anxiously for the pregnancy test. It was positive! We were elated but cautious, since we'd had so many pregnancy losses. Our surrogate went for her first ultrasound and then called and asked me if I was sitting down. I was petrified of bad news—had she miscarried? Instead, the news was that we were pregnant with twins. I screamed with joy.

Now I had to face the reality of a twin pregnancy and all the risks associated with it. Would the pregnancy go to term and result in delivery of healthy babies? Would our surrogate follow recommendations of bed rest, if needed? I knew once we got past 32 weeks it would probably be okay. It was getting to that mark that was hard. In the end we made it to 38 weeks and a Cesarean section was scheduled because the babies were breech. We flew to California for the birth and became the proud parents of twin girls. Our lives were forever changed. I am so grateful that someone would be so giving of herself as to carry my children. There is a special place in heaven for our surrogate and all the women who reach beyond themselves and selflessly give to others.

Chapter 7

DOMESTIC AND INTERNATIONAL ADOPTIONS

Adopting a child, whether newborn or older, within the United States or internationally, can be an exciting and fulfilling way to create or add to your family. Many different types of adoption are available for you to consider, although figuring them out and deciding which one to pursue can be confusing because there are so many labels. In this chapter, we describe the four basic types of adoption: domestic public agency adoption, domestic private agency adoption, domestic independent adoption, and international adoption. Most people have also heard the terms "open adoption" and "closed adoption." An open adoption is one in which the birth parents and adoptive parents share information or have contact with each other before, during, or after a child's adoption. In a closed adoption no information is shared. Open adoptions can range from confidential, in which minimal information is shared and a third party, such as an agency, transmits the information, to fully disclosed, in which all relevant information is shared and adoptive and birth families may even have face-to-face meetings and ongoing contact after birth.

DOMESTIC PUBLIC AGENCY ADOPTIONS

Public adoption agencies are usually part of a state's social services department. Most states operate several adoption agencies, on either a regional or a national level. To find a public agency, look in the yellow pages section of the telephone book under "Department of Social Services" or "Department of Public Welfare."

The public adoption agencies primarily place children who have been in the foster care system. Some of the children in foster care have special needs, including both physical and psychological needs, but other children have no physical health problems. Children in the foster care system have been taken from unfit homes and placed into foster homes for a time. Their biological parents' rights have usually been involuntarily terminated (or are in the process of being terminated) because of abuse or neglect. The length of time that a child stays in a foster home varies. Depending on the state, the average time in foster care can range from 9 to 38 months.

Most of the children available for adoption through a state foster care system are classified as "older," which means they can be as young as two years and as old as seventeen. Preschoolers (children five years and under) are the age group most likely to be adopted. Many of the foster care children awaiting adoption placement are children of color. Many public agencies only accept adoption applications from families wanting to adopt older children, sibling groups, or children with special needs.

Foster parenting is a possible route to adoption. Although public child welfare agencies are committed to trying to return children to their birth families, there is a growing trend toward freeing foster children for adoption (that is, terminating the parental rights of the birth parents) as quickly as possible. Recent federal legislation has mandated courts to seek termination of parental rights when a child has been in foster care for 15 of the last 22 months, unless there are extenuating circumstances. Some states have begun to consider foster parenting and adoption as a continuum rather than two different functions. In states where foster parenting can lead to adoption, a public adoption agency may ask applicants if they want to be only foster parents, only adoptive parents, or foster/adoptive parents. If applicants choose to be foster/adoptive parents and the child they foster is freed for adoption, they may be given priority consideration as the potential adoptive parents.

Public agencies have two advantages over other pathways to adoption: they are less expensive and child placement occurs quickly. If you decide to pursue a public agency adoption, you will need to have a home study (as with any adoption) and also take classes to qualify as an adoptive parent. You can also expect frequent home inspections and supervision from social workers immediately following the adoption. The subsequent frequency and duration of the visits will depend on your situation. Adoptions from foster care are usually closed adoptions, but an adoption agency may offer other options.

The basic steps you can expect to follow if you pursue a domestic adoption through a public agency are as follows:

1. You submit an application to the agency of your choice, and if accepted into the program, you are charged an initial fee. Applications are usually accepted or denied within 60 days.
2. You undergo a home study (discussed in chapter 15).
3. You are placed on a waiting list, and when a child becomes available, you can decide to accept or turn down the proposed child.
4. Once you accept a proposed child, the child comes to live with you. During this postplacement period, the agency social worker makes several visits to monitor the child's progress.
5. The agency usually recommends that adoption be granted six months after the child's placement with you, at which point the local court is allowed to finalize the adoption.
6. Finalizing the adoption involves a judicial proceeding in court or in the judge's chambers. The proceeding is attended by the adoptive parent or parents, the child to be adopted, the adoptive family's attorney, and the agency social worker who placed the child.

DOMESTIC PRIVATE AGENCY ADOPTIONS

Private adoption agencies mainly work with people wanting to adopt an infant at birth or as soon after birth as possible. Private agencies operate as either for-profit or nonprofit organizations, but there is little difference between the two types for prospective adoptive parents. The fees and adoption process are essentially the same. All private agencies must be licensed by the state, and they are licensed to offer specific services. The scope of services offered varies; some agencies are only licensed to conduct home studies, whereas others are licensed as full-service adoption agencies.

Private agencies may keep a waiting list of people wanting to adopt and go to the next person or couple on the list when a child becomes available. More often, though, an agency tries to match a child with adoptive parents who can most effectively meet the child's needs. The characteristics that would be considered are the prospective parents' readiness to adopt, their financial status, how well their ethnicity and physical appearance match the child's, and their religious affiliation.

The waiting time can be long—as long as several years for a newborn Caucasian baby—if the agency looks for a birth mother. To decrease the waiting time, some agencies allow prospective parents to search for a birth mother. In these cases, called identified or designated agency adoptions, the agency facilitates the adoption process but does not find the birth mother. The prospective parents take care of the advertising, and the advertisement requests that the birth mother call the agency directly. Identified adoptions can also occur when a birth mother has already made an agreement with the adoptive parents before involving an agency. An identified adoption proceeds like an independent adoption (discussed later in this chapter), except that an agency is involved to provide guidance, and the laws governing an agency adoption are followed rather than those governing an independent adoption. For an identified adoption, the agency may or may not name an attorney; if not, the adoptive parents must find an attorney themselves.

Private agencies offer both closed and open adoptions. Traditionally, adoptions have been closed, meaning that the birth parents and adoptive parents never meet or share information. In this scenario, an agency calls the prospective parents, who have completed all the necessary steps for adoption, to say that a baby is available and has been released for adoption. The baby may be a newborn, whom the adoptive parents pick up from the hospital, or the baby may have been in foster care for a few weeks. Depending on the state, the birth mother may be allowed a set period of time—anywhere from a few days to 90 days—to change her mind after the baby's birth. Some agencies will not permit a child to be placed in an adoptive home before the waiting period has ended, and in some states it is illegal to place a child before the waiting period has ended.

Today, the trend is moving away from closed adoptions toward open adoptions. In most private agency adoptions, the birth mother and the adoptive parents meet prior to the birth. Many adoptive parents are able to be present at the birth, and once the biological mother signs the papers relinquishing the baby, they may be able to take the baby home from the hospital. Depending on the state, though, the baby may be taken by the agency for the duration of the waiting period and then released to the adoptive parents. The adoptive parents and the birth mother or birth parents maintain an open line of communication after the adoption has been finalized. Open adoption scenarios range from exchanging photos once a year to getting together for special occasions.

Regardless of whether a private agency adoption is open or closed, the prospective parents pay the birth mother's legal, living, counseling, and medical (if the birth mother has no insurance) expenses in addition to the agency fee. Living expenses generally start when the birth mother agrees to the adoption. Some agencies receive outside funds and can subsidize the cost to prospective parents.

If you pursue a domestic private agency adoption, the process will most likely follow these steps:

1. You submit an application to the agency of your choice, and if accepted into the program, you are charged an initial fee. Applications are usually accepted or denied within 60 days.

2. You may be asked to provide a portfolio with photos and information for birth mothers to look through, and you may need to write a "Dear Birth Mother" letter.
3. You complete a home study (discussed in chapter 15).
4. The agency identifies birth mothers through outreach and advertising and provides them with counseling sessions.
5. The agency contacts you once a potential birth mother has been identified, and you have the option to refuse that particular birth mother. If you accept the birth mother and the adoption is to be open, you will meet the birth mother.
6. The birth mother delivers the baby, and you take the baby home either from the hospital or at the end of the waiting period.
7. The agency social worker makes several postplacement visits to monitor the baby's progress.
8. The agency usually recommends that adoption be granted six months after the baby's placement with you, at which point the local court is allowed to finalize the adoption.
9. Finalizing the adoption involves a judicial proceeding in court or in the judge's chambers. The proceeding is attended by the adoptive parent or parents, the child to be adopted, the adoptive family's attorney, and the agency social worker who placed the child.

DOMESTIC INDEPENDENT ADOPTIONS

Independent adoptions (also called nonagency, private, or self-directed adoptions) proceed without using the services of an agency. If you decide to follow this route, you will need to hire an attorney who either locates a birth mother for you or instructs you on how to find one yourself through advertising or networking. To show the birth mother what type of life you can offer as adoptive parents, you need to put together a portfolio and write a "Dear Birth Mother" letter.

Only 1 in 10 birth mothers who intend to place their child for adoption go through with relinquishing their child, so be prepared for the possibility of a birth mother changing her mind. Because an agency is not involved, you and your lawyer handle all aspects of the adoption process and maintain communications with the birth mother throughout the pregnancy and potentially following birth. In independent adoptions, the adoptive parents generally cover minimal living expenses for the birth mother, as well as medical care if she is uninsured (additional information on costs is given in chapter 16).

INTERNATIONAL ADOPTIONS

Adopting a child from another country has grown in popularity in the past decade. Many prospective parents opt for an international adoption because the wait is relatively short and predictable, they do not need to "sell" themselves to a birth mother, and the risk of adoption disruption is minimal. Children available for international adoption are classified as orphans and are freed for adoption in their home countries. These children have been placed in orphanages or foster homes in their country because the birth parents have died, relinquished their parental rights, or had their rights terminated by abandoning the child. Every country has its own laws, regulations, restrictions, and eligibility requirements.

The process begins with selecting a country from which to adopt, working with an agency or lawyer, and filling out a substantial amount of paperwork—termed a petition—to file with the agency and the U.S. Immigration and Naturalization Service (INS). Prospective parents also need to have an approved home study completed by a licensed social worker. If the petition is approved by the INS and a child has been identified, the INS notifies the U.S. embassy or consulate in the child's country. A copy of the petition is sent with accompanying documentation to the National Visa Center, where it is assigned a computer tracking code. Once a visa has been issued for the child, the adoptive parents can travel to the child's country to get the child. If a child has not yet been identified, the petition is sent to the U.S. embassy in the country that the prospective parents plan to adopt from, and the couple waits for a child to be identified.

Although independent or nonagency international adoptions are possible, the vast majority of these adoptions occur through agencies experienced in international adoptions. An agency deals with the logistics of an international adoption, which for most people are simply too bewildering and time-consuming. Agencies are also familiar with the protocol required in the particular country. Adoptive parents generally need to make one or two trips abroad (see chapter 14). The agency makes the travel arrangements, including arranging for guides and translators. Depending on the country they decide to adopt from, prospective parents may receive videotapes of the child before traveling, or they may see the child for the first time on a visit to the country. While in the country, prospective parents will meet the child at the orphanage or foster home, and they may be taken on trips to experience and learn something about the country's culture. They may also be expected to appear in court once or twice for a preliminary hearing and to finalize the adoption. Chapter 14 gives some more details on international adoptions.

The adoption laws and regulations of the country in which the child was born guide international adoptions. The courts or a similar government body in the birth country usually handle the legal matters, and neither the U.S. government nor the INS can intervene with the proceedings.

The top 10 countries for international adoptions in fiscal year 2005 (ending September 30, 2005) are shown in table 7.1. The total number of international adoptions in 2005, estimated from immigrant visas issued to orphans coming to the United States, was 22,728 (http://adoption.about.com/od/statistic1/f/2005visas.htm).

Table 7.1. Countries with the Highest Numbers of Children Adopted to the United States in 2005

Country	Number of adoptions
China (mainland)	7,906
Russia	4,639
Guatemala	3,783
South Korea	1,630
Ukraine	821
Kazakhstan	755
Ethiopia	441
India	323
Colombia	291
Philippines	271

FURTHER READING

L. Beauvais-Godwin and R. Godwin. *Complete Adoption Book: Everything You Need to Know to Adopt a Child.* Adams Media, 2000.

J. N. Erichsen and H. R. Erichsen. *How to Adopt Internationally: A Guide for Agency-Directed and Independent Adoptions.* Mesa House, 2003.

R. Mintzer. *Yes, You Can Adopt! A Comprehensive Guide to Adoption.* Avalon, Carroll and Graf, 2003.

O. R. Sweet and P. Bryan. *Adopt International: Everything You Need to Know to Adopt a Child from Abroad.* Noonday Press, 1996.

WHEN I LEFT A MARRIAGE that didn't work, I had already decided that I didn't want marriage or any partnership. I was independent and self-reliant, I enjoyed my work, and I loved living alone in my own house. But I had a quandary: I wanted to be a mom. How was I to have a child without a partner? I spent a couple of years reading and pondering the many methods available to make a baby. In the end, I realized I was not willing to undergo any of these procedures. They were somehow too invasive, and the thought of mixing my genes with those of an unknown male donor was rather distasteful to me. I would rather look into my child's eyes and see her as an individual and not be wondering whether or not she takes after my family or the stranger who provided the other half of her genes. That's when I realized that being a mom was more important than procreating. After a trip to Africa brought home to me the reality of poverty and loss in the world, I also realized that there were already lots of babies in the world who desperately needed a family. So there it was, adoption was the answer. I could be a mom and do my part to make a child's life one of security and opportunity, enriched by the love I had to give.

I chose an international adoption because at that time it was the quickest way to bring a child into my family. It took a year before I brought home my beautiful baby daughter. Amazingly, four years later I found myself adopting again. So now here I am, a single, working parent to two gorgeous girls who are eight and twelve years old. It's hard (sometimes very hard) being a single, working parent, but I have never had one moment of regret. This was what I was meant to do. I am deeply grateful to be living in a country that accepts and is supportive of single parents and racially mixed families.

Chapter 8

WHICH OPTIONS ARE AVAILABLE TO YOU?

The Requirements for Each Pathway

In the previous chapters, we've outlined the basic process that occurs with each of the available options for fertility assistance, surrogacy, and adoption. Now that you're familiar with the options, you will want to determine which ones are available to you, given your circumstances. If you are healthy, wealthy, and young, and have been happily married for several years, all or most of the possibilities should be available to you and your partner. Few people fit this description, though, so don't be disheartened! You still have a variety of options.

The characteristics most likely to limit your options are age, marital status, financial resources, and underlying medical conditions. Extremes within these characteristics will eliminate certain options, but, almost always, another is available. For example, a fifty-year-old single woman would be unable to use her own eggs for fertility assistance, but she could pursue an independent domestic adoption or an international adoption from some countries (although because of her age she may not be eligible to adopt a very young child). She may also be a candidate for donor eggs.

Throughout this chapter, we describe the general eligibility requirements for each of the pathways to parenthood. Chapter 9 discusses the challenges for nontraditional families, including singles, cohabitating heterosexual couples, and same-sex couples, and for people with specific conditions such as human immunodeficiency virus (HIV) infection.

FERTILITY ASSISTANCE

Most healthy individuals qualify for the initial fertility evaluations and early fertility assistance. With more invasive and intensive assisted reproductive technology (ART) procedures, a woman's or a couple's eligibility depends on the initial evaluation, prior fertility assistance attempts, age, and additional testing. Testing may identify medical conditions that could disqualify a woman or a couple from using ART. ART methods are also expensive and are often not covered by insurance, so these factors may restrict some people from being able to try them. Physical and medical conditions that commonly restrict people's use of ART methods, whether using their own eggs or donor eggs, are listed in table 8.1.

Abnormalities of the uterus can cause infertility and are also associated with recurrent miscarriages. A very common uterine problem is the presence of fibroids. Uterine fibroids are tumors or growths made up of muscle cells and other tissues that grow within the wall of the uterus. Even though fibroids are called tumors, they are almost always benign (not cancerous). Because fibroids are located in the uterine wall, they can interfere with the implantation of an embryo. Problems with an embryo implanting also occur in women with scar tissue inside the uterus and in women with an abnormally shaped uterus. If you are trying to become pregnant and have a uterine abnormality, your doctor will discuss with you whether or not you need to be treated and what the treatment options are.

An ultrasound of the ovaries can reveal abnormalities such as ovarian cysts. An ovarian cyst is a collection of fluid surrounding an egg in the ovary. Ovarian cysts don't usually cause fertility prob-

Table 8.1. Physical and Medical Conditions That Restrict Use of Assisted Reproductive Technology

---

- Selected infections, including human immunodeficiency virus (HIV) infection[1] and active hepatitis C infection
- Abnormal uterus[2]
- Abnormal body mass index (very underweight or overweight)
- Age[3]

Restrictions for women using their own eggs

- Starting menopause, poor "ovarian reserve" (ovary is showing the effect of mother's age, as determined by blood testing)
- Abnormal ultrasound of ovaries[4]

Restriction for male partner

- No sperm

---

1. Some programs will do in vitro fertilization if testing shows the level of HIV to be so low that it can't be detected by current laboratory methods. European centers are generally more liberal than U.S. centers.

2. Women with an abnormal uterus still have the option of using their own eggs in a surrogacy arrangement. Uterine diseases are discussed later in this chapter.

3. Most programs do not have an age limit for women using their own eggs, as long as they have not gone through menopause. However, the chances of success are low with maternal age over 40, as discussed later in this chapter. The age limit for women using donor eggs is usually between 52 and 60 years.

4. Ovarian diseases are discussed later in this chapter.

lems, but some women, particularly if they have large cysts, experience bleeding and pain. The issue for fertility assistance is that hormone stimulation can cause an ovarian cyst to grow larger, which may cause problems for women who already have large cysts at the outset of their fertility treatment. Occasionally, an ovarian ultrasound suggests that cancerous tissue may be present in the ovary. In this case, the woman is immediately referred for further tests to find out if the ovary is indeed cancerous and how best to deal with it.

The initial fertility workup might indicate that, even with fertility treatments, some women or couples have extremely low chances—less than 1 percent—for a successful pregnancy. Fertility specialists may refuse to offer treatment to women or couples with such a poor prognosis, but the specialist should still thoroughly discuss treatment decisions and, ideally, will suggest other options.

People with disabilities or certain medical conditions may worry that a fertility center will not accept them as patients. Nobody should be denied fertility treatment solely because of a disability. People with specific blood infections, such as hepatitis or HIV, also have options, including fertility assistance, to become parents. Chapter 9 includes specific information for people with blood infections. Sometimes, a fertility program decides not to offer services to an individual or couple on the basis of a "well-substantiated" judgment that they either cannot provide for a child or would not be adequate parents.

Using Your Own Eggs

A single factor is, overwhelmingly, the most likely to determine whether a woman has the option of using her own eggs: her age. As shown in table 8.2, women have increasing difficulty in achieving a successful pregnancy outcome as they approach forty years old. The older a woman, the more likely it is that her eggs will have chromosomal abnormalities; as a result, miscarriage rates increase with age.

Maternal age remains a critical factor for women who seek fertility assistance. As women get older, they have increasing difficulty at every step in the process of conceiving a child:

- An older woman is less likely to respond successfully to hormone stimulation and less likely to progress to egg retrieval.
- A cycle that progresses to egg retrieval is slightly less likely to reach the embryo transfer stage.
- A cycle that progresses to embryo transfer is less likely to continue to pregnancy.
- A cycle that progresses to pregnancy is less likely to result in a live birth, because of the greater risk of miscarriage in older women. The 2003 figures published by the Centers for Disease Control for miscarriage rates in ART cycles were less than 13 percent per cycle for women younger than thirty-

four years, 29 percent at age forty, and 43 percent at age forty-three.

Using Your Own Sperm

Except in a condition called azoospermia, in which a man's body does not make sperm, most men can use their own sperm in assisted fertility procedures. Men with very low levels of sperm can be helped by a procedure called intracytoplasmic sperm injection (ICSI). For a fertility center to use the ICSI technique, a sperm sample only needs to contain one live sperm. As described in chapter 3, ICSI is a laboratory procedure used with ART for couples who are having difficulty conceiving in part because of male factor infertility. ICSI can be used to bypass a variety of problems with the man's sperm:

- The sperm sample has a very low number of sperm with normal movement (a condition called teratospermia).
- The sperm have difficulty binding to and penetrating the egg.

Table 8.2. Effect of Maternal Age on Conception, Chromosomal Abnormalities, and Miscarriage

Maternal age in years	Not conceiving after trying for one year	Chromosomal abnormalities	Miscarriages
<30	1/5 (20%)	1/526 (0.2%)	1/6.7 (15%)
30–35	1/5 (20%)	1/385 (0.3%)	1/6.7 (15%)
36–40	1/3 (33%)	1/192 (0.5%)	1/5.9 (17%)
41–45	2/3 (66%)	1/66 (1.5%)	1/2.9 (34%)
>45	95/100 (95%)	1/21 (5%)	1/1.9 (53%)

Source: Adapted from J. Meyers-Thompson and S. Perkins. *Fertility for Dummies.* New York: Wiley Publishing, © 2003, p. 9.

- The woman's body reacts to the sperm by making anti-sperm antibodies that can destroy the sperm.
- Fertilization of the woman's eggs has been unsuccessful in earlier attempts with standard in vitro fertilization (IVF).
- The sperm sample contains a limited number of good-quality sperm.
- An obstruction of the male reproductive tract prevents sperm from entering the ejaculate and the obstruction cannot be repaired (in this case, sperm can be harvested directly from the testicles).

For a man's sperm to be used in an ART procedure, he must be clear of sexually transmitted infections such as gonorrhea and chlamydia. Men with chronic infections, including HIV and hepatitis, are able to use their own sperm in some situations; these are discussed in chapter 9.

Using Donor Sperm, Eggs, or Embryos

Most women, with or without a partner, are eligible for donor sperm, eggs, and embryos. The only real criteria are that the woman should be healthy and should not have a medical condition that could jeopardize the pregnancy. However, for a woman to be a donor egg or embryo recipient, most fertility centers usually require at least one prior IVF attempt, except in specific cases (if, for example, the woman has an inheritable condition that prohibits using her own eggs or she has already gone through menopause). Some centers require a couple to be married to be eligible for donor eggs or embryos. Donor programs generally have a maternal age requirement for recipients (no older than fifty-two to sixty years, on average), but the recipient need not be pre-menopausal. In fact, many older recipients of donor eggs are candidates precisely because their age and menopause have caused their infertility.

Couples who donate embryos are able to add criteria of their own for the individual or couple receiving the embryos. For example, couples can choose to donate only to people of a specific religion. They can also specify that recipients receive counseling, and they can choose to maintain contact after birth.

SURROGACY

Over the last 10 years, surrogacy programs have become much more liberal in their criteria for people who want to use a surrogate. They are generally open to working with diverse groups, including same-sex couples and single women. The individual or couple wishing to use a surrogate (sometimes called the commissioning individual or couple) should be in good physical and mental health and may be required to undergo physical examinations and psychological evaluations. The man who donates the sperm will need to undergo screening for sexually transmitted diseases and possibly have a consultation with a geneticist.

Women for whom surrogacy is one of the last available options generally fall into one of three medical categories:

1. Their ovaries function but not their uterus, because of a congenital condition, because they have had a hysterectomy, or for other medical reasons.
2. They have had repeated miscarriages and the possibility of carrying a baby to term is remote, or they have been unable to conceive with other assisted reproductive methods.
3. They have a medical condition that makes pregnancy life-threatening, but they are otherwise healthy.

Other types of individuals and couples may also seek surrogacy services. Couples who have been unsuccessful after several IVF attempts, even though the embryos appear healthy and the woman's uterus seems to be normal, may want to try surrogacy. Some physicians believe that for couples in this situation, a gestational carrier may offer a chance for success. However, other physicians are uncertain about the chance of success even with a gestational carrier, so there is some controversy about recommending surrogacy for these couples. A gay male couple may also decide to pursue a surrogacy arrangement.

The United States does not regulate surrogacy, but a few individual states have their own laws. For example, in Florida, surrogacy is only allowed if the commissioning mother cannot physically carry a pregnancy to term. Legal issues surrounding surrogacy are discussed in chapters 6 and 17.

ADOPTION

People who want to adopt a child must meet a variety of requirements, some of which depend on the type of adoption. In general, though, there are certain basic characteristics that all adoptive parents must have, regardless of the type of adoption they intend to pursue. When an agency is involved, the agency usually uses information supplied on the application and during the home study to establish whether an individual or a couple has these necessary characteristics. Applicants must demonstrate the following:

- They are stable and loving people.
- They are healthy enough to meet a child's needs.
- They have a normal life expectancy.
- They have sufficient income to provide for a child.
- They have adequate space for a child to live in (but it is not necessary to own a home).
- If married, they have a healthy marriage.
- If already parents, they have children who do not exhibit problems related to poor parenting.
- They don't have an extensive divorce history.
- They don't have a history of mental illness, criminal activity, child abuse, or drug or alcohol addiction.

Every person or couple who applies to adopt must complete a home study, and then must be recommended by the social worker who conducted the study as suitable to be adoptive parents. In addition to assessing the basic characteristics listed above, a home study may include other items. The regulations about the extent of a home study are established by each state. Home studies for public agencies may be more demanding than those for private agencies, because children being adopted through a public agency are more likely to have disabilities and special needs. Further information about home studies is included in chapter 15.

Domestic Agency Adoption

In addition to the basic characteristics that applicants must meet, most public and private agencies have specific requirements that can relate to one or more of several other factors: age, religion, weight, ethnic background, income, educational level, medical condition, marital status, and infertility diagnosis. Many agencies typically have the following additional requirements for people who want to adopt:

- They must be no more than forty years older than the child they are adopting.
- If married, they must have been married for at least three years. (Singles are usually allowed to adopt, particularly special needs children.)
- They must be medically unable to conceive a child or must be able to show that it is unsafe for them to conceive a child.
- They must have no more than one child already.

Religious affiliation can facilitate or hinder adoption efforts; some agencies will only work with prospective parents from specific religious backgrounds.

For people interested in adopting a special needs child, a public agency may waive some of its usual requirements regarding age, marital status, fertility status, and existing children. In particular, single people often find it easiest to adopt a child who has been in foster care. According to the U.S. Department of Health and Human Services, one in three children adopted from foster care is adopted by a single parent. Some states report that one of every five agency adoptions is by a single parent.

Domestic Independent Adoption

Most people are eligible to pursue an independent adoption, unless they live in a state where independent adoptions are illegal. The restrictions imposed by agencies don't apply, so, in general, the only requirement is to meet the list of basic characteristics, which are determined during the home study.

International Adoption

Each country specifies the criteria for adoptive parents. These criteria are generally more liberal than those specified by public agencies for domestic adoptions. The acceptable average age of the prospective parent is higher, and single people are often eligible. Some countries will not allow lesbian or gay couples to adopt. The criteria for the most popular countries participating in international adoptions, as of the time of writing this book, are shown in table 8.3.

FURTHER READING

L. Beauvais-Godwin and R. Godwin. *Complete Adoption Book: Everything You Need to Know to Adopt a Child.* Adams Media, 2000.

J. N. Erichsen and H. R. Erichsen. *How to Adopt Internationally: A Guide for Agency-Directed and Independent Adoptions.* Mesa House, 2003.

J. Meyers-Thompson and S. Perkins. *Fertility for Dummies.* Wiley, 2003.

R. Mintzer. *Yes, You Can Adopt! A Comprehensive Guide to Adoption.* Avalon, Carroll and Graf, 2003.

G. Sutton. *A Matter of Trust: The Guide to Gestational Surrogacy.* Clouds Publishing, 1997.

O. R. Sweet and P. Bryan. *Adopt International: Everything You Need to Know to Adopt a Child from Abroad.* Noonday Press, 1996.

Table 8.3. Common Requirements for International Adoption from Ten Countries

Country	Age in years[1]	Singles	Length of marriage in years
China	>29	Heterosexual persons[2]	—
Russia	>24; <46 years older than child	Yes	—
Guatemala	25–55	Yes	>2
South Korea	25–44	No	>2
Ukraine	>18; >15 years older than child	Yes	—
Kazakhstan	>16 years older than child	Yes	—
Ethiopia	<41 years older than child	Heterosexual women >25 years old[2]	>4
India	—	Women only	—
Colombia	>25	Can adopt children >7 years old	—
Philippines	>26; >15 years older than child	—	>2

1. Applicants aged 30 to 45 years can expect a referral of a child 6 to 18 months old; applicants aged 46 to 50 can expect a child 14 to 30 months old; and applicants over 50 should be open to a child from 30 months to 5 years old. For a married couple to adopt, as long as one spouse is under 54 years old, the other spouse can be any age over 29 years.

2. Both China and Ethiopia prohibit gay and lesbian adoptions.

I AM FORTY YEARS OLD and single. I have a successful career, and until recent years I was happy with where I was in life, except I wanted children more than anything. My biological clock was ticking with a vengeance! Where was Mr. Right? I was dating a great guy, but he refused to commit to marriage and parenthood. He wouldn't even forgo the marriage and just agree to parenthood. I didn't know what to do. Should I stop taking my pills and get pregnant whether he liked it or not? Should I end the relationship and try to find a partner who wanted children? Should I just go to a fertility clinic and select donor sperm?

I chose to proceed with donor sperm. At the initial visit I was given information on sperm bank programs. I had to choose my future child's father from a catalog. It took a little while to get over what a nonintimate process I was going to embark upon. I selected a donor and the specimens were shipped to the clinic. After all infectious disease screens and consultations were complete, I underwent insemination. The insemination was very simple. It was like having a Pap smear in the gynecologist's office. I waited two weeks and found out I wasn't pregnant.

It took five attempts and the addition of fertility medications to get pregnant. Finally I did, and I delivered a healthy baby boy. Life is wonderful! My partner became distant during my pregnancy and our relationship ended. Single parenting is not an easy job, but for me, it is certainly worth it.

Chapter 9

CONSIDERATIONS FOR

NONTRADITIONAL FAMILIES

Some people want very much to raise a child but find themselves in a situation or with a medical condition that limits their options for fertility assistance, surrogacy, or adoption. The challenges for people who are single, unmarried, gay or lesbian, or affected by a blood infection are often greater than for married heterosexual couples, but they are by no means insurmountable. Options exist for every one of these groups of people to welcome a child into their family.

SINGLES

The 2000 Census estimates that approximately 12 million households in the United States are single-parent homes. A single woman can pursue parenthood through sperm donation, assistance at a fertility center, or adoption. A single man can consider surrogacy or adoption.

Single-parent adoption has become increasingly popular and is easier than in the past. Single adoptive parents are more likely to adopt older children and special needs children, and they are less likely to have been a foster parent to the adopted child. More than one million single fathers live in the United States, but most single adoptive parents are women. Single men have many barriers to overcome when dealing with birth mothers or adoption agencies. These barriers include the perceived need for a mother, issues with the lifestyle of single men, and concerns about child molestation. Nevertheless, a single man is still able to adopt, particularly if he would like to adopt an older boy, at least five years old.

Some studies have shown that children raised in single-parent homes have higher rates of depression, drug abuse, teen pregnancy, and other difficulties than children living in an intact two-parent home. However, many of these same studies have also found that the children's problems were probably due in part to other factors such as depression in the custodial parent or parents, parental conflicts, emotional trauma due to separation and disruption, and financial difficulties. Most experts would probably agree that children brought up in a stable, loving environment will thrive regardless of how many parents are active in the children's lives.

People interested in being a single parent need to realize that both becoming a parent and raising a child may be harder because of their single status. If you decide to pursue single parenting, you should consider or at least be aware of the possible emotional, logistical, and financial difficulties:

- Friends, family, and others may be critical of you for parenting a child on your own.
- If you decide to try fertility assistance or to adopt, you may need to explain how you will manage as a single parent.
- You will need to explain to your child at some point why he or she has only one parent.
- Your dating life and potential for a partner relationship may be greatly affected.
- You shoulder all the time commitment and the entire financial burden.
- Birth mothers may prefer a couple.
- Some adoption agencies will not accept applications from single parents.
- Several countries do not allow single-parent adoption, and others make it difficult.

On the other hand, there are positive aspects to being a single parent. A single parent makes all the parenting decisions, which can make life easier than for two parents who are unable to agree on certain issues. A variety of resources are available to single parents, such as the organization Single Mothers by Choice.

UNMARRIED COHABITING
HETEROSEXUAL COUPLES

People who are unmarried and living together as heterosexual partners generally need to work as a couple in pursuing parenthood. The first thing that each partner in the relationship should consider is that he or she will be co-parenting with the other partner for the next 18 years. Married or not, the partners will be bound to each other.

Most fertility centers will work with unmarried couples, although some centers require couples to be married if they want to use donor egg services. If partners are not married because of a relationship problem, they may be putting themselves in a vulnerable position during the time of fertility assistance, which can consume months to years. For example, just waiting for donor eggs can take several months, and only then do the attempts at pregnancy begin. Once committed to using assisted reproductive technology (ART), it is difficult to consider stopping part way through a cycle or after one unsuccessful attempt. Some people find themselves tolerating a bad relationship in an attempt to achieve pregnancy. If you are unsure about your relationship, consider how you will cope with a child—for your sake and the child's sake—before you make the emotional and financial commitment.

An unmarried couple may have limited options if they want to adopt a child, whether domestically or internationally. Technically, one partner could apply to adopt as a single individual, but the home study would reflect the shared living arrangement and the application might be denied on this basis. The home study is less stringent for nonagency or independent adoptions, yet an unmarried couple still needs to give a good explanation for not being married to put themselves in the best light. Questions to expect during the home study include, Are you not ready to be married? Is your partner not the right person? Is it that you don't want to be alone but haven't yet found the right person? Do you think your partner will be a bad parent?

Some states issue a Certificate of Informal Marriage to couples who qualify according to common-law marriage guidelines. The partners must prove, through paid receipts, when they began living together and first presented themselves as married. This certificate is accepted by some, but not all, courts abroad. If you apply for an international adoption, ask the agency if the certificate is accepted by the country you're interested in. The certificate may also be accepted by some domestic agencies.

LESBIAN AND GAY COUPLES

Of the more than 600,000 gay and lesbian couples living together in the United States, according to the 2000 Census, about 60,000 male couples and 96,000 female couples have at least one child under eighteen years of age living at home. The Human Rights Campaign, a gay rights group, believes the number of same-sex couples with children is considerably higher. Children of Lesbians and Gays Everywhere (COLAGE) is one of several national support groups geared to the estimated 250,000 children of gay and lesbian couples and the millions of other children who have a gay parent. Gay parent magazines provide resources on gay-friendly private schools, camps, and vacations, and there are several children's books about growing up with gay parents.

Although most research has been done on lesbian couples, all studies conclude that the stability of the parents' relationship—not their sexual orientation—determines the quality of the child's upbringing. But there are some differences. Boys raised by same-sex parents tend to be less aggressive, more nurturing, and more sexually restrained than those raised in heterosexual families. Girls raised by same-sex parents tend to be more sexually adventurous and self-confident. Opponents of same-sex parenting argue that a major problem is depriving a child of an opposite-sex parent, but this argument may be more of a cultural than a scientific one.

As of 2003, gays and lesbians were allowed to adopt in every state except Florida, Mississippi, and Utah. If a gay or lesbian couple wants to adopt a baby at birth, they may worry about whether or not a birth mother would choose them over a heterosexual couple. Some birth mothers, though, may feel more comfortable placing their child with two women than with a man and woman. Also, the strength of gay and lesbian couples to stand up and not hide who they are can appeal to some birth mothers.

International adoptions can be more difficult for gays and lesbians, depending on the country that interests them. Some countries will only place a child with an adoptive parent or parents who convince the authorities of their heterosexuality with a written statement. In other words, gays and lesbians would have to deny their sexual orientation and state that they are heterosexual. Some lesbian or gay couples may try to adopt by having only one partner apply as a single parent and by not disclosing information about their sexuality—the "don't ask, don't tell" policy. However, as with unmarried cohabiting heterosexual couples who attempt to mask their living arrangement, the home study will most likely reveal the situation.

Partners in gay and lesbian relationships may have more difficulty than heterosexual partners in achieving custodial rights to their child, unless both partners are named as the child's legal parents. Unless both are the legal parents, if the couple splits up or something happens to one partner, a family member may sue for custody, resulting in a court battle. Similarly, a lesbian couple who achieve parenthood through fertility assistance may face custodial issues, depending on who donated the egg and who carried the pregnancy. Unless both women are legally the parents, if the relationship ends, one woman may lose custody. The same issue could be faced by a gay couple if one man donated the sperm for a surrogate pregnancy. Some experts think that the safest route in protecting parental rights is for both partners to legally adopt the child, regardless of whether the child is genetically related to one or to neither parent.

PEOPLE WITH A BLOOD INFECTION

Many people who have a blood-borne infection such as HIV/ AIDS, hepatitis B, or hepatitis C can become parents, despite their infection. Appropriate medical and obstetrical care for the mother and infant can reduce the risks of both partner-to-partner transmission and mother-to-child transmission. Adoption is also a possibility for people with blood infections. The Americans with Disabilities Act (ADA) gives federal civil rights protection to individuals with disabilities, including people with HIV/AIDS or hepatitis. One ADA provision is that adoption agencies may not use "standards or criteria or methods of discrimination that have the effect of discriminating on the basis of disability" (www .cwla.org/programs/adoption/Americans_with_disabilities.htm). Therefore, adoption agencies cannot categorically reject applicants based on their HIV or hepatitis status.

HIV/AIDS and hepatitis are discussed separately below.

HIV/AIDS

Discordant couples—where one partner has HIV and the other doesn't—have several options for becoming pregnant, depending on which partner is infected. Even when both partners have HIV, they should not be exposed to each other's virus, because one strain may be more virulent. To minimize the transmission risk, they should follow the strategies outlined below for discordant couples.

When only the female partner has HIV, the transmission risk to her male partner can be eliminated by using insemination techniques. The simplest way is for the man or woman to insert the sperm into the woman's vagina at home using a syringe (without the needle). The couple can also go to a fertility clinic for intracervical insemination (ICI) or intrauterine insemination (IUI), in which the sperm are inserted with a small tube directly into the cervix or uterus (see chapters 2 and 4). With these techniques, the male partner is not at risk for catching HIV, but the female partner could catch other sexually transmitted infections from the man.

For discordant couples in which the male partner has HIV, the transmission rate is estimated to be approximately 1 in every 500 to 1,000 episodes of unprotected intercourse. The transmission rate can be decreased, but the risk cannot be eliminated, by using HIV treatments to lower the amount of virus in the blood and semen. HIV/AIDS drug treatments can decrease both the blood and semen HIV to extremely low levels, to the point of being undetectable. Fertility centers also offer sperm washing, a technique that separates the sperm from the fluid parts of the semen. The fluid in the semen is more likely to contain HIV than are the actual sperm cells. The washed sperm can be checked for HIV and not used for insemination if the virus remains. A third option to minimize the risk of transmission from an infected man to his uninfected female partner is the use of IVF treatment with intracytoplasmic sperm injection (ICSI). With this technique, the woman is only exposed to the single sperm cell injected into the egg. ICSI is described in more detail in chapter 3.

Some states have made it illegal for tissue of any kind (including sperm and semen) to be donated by an HIV-infected person. In these states, therefore, a woman cannot be inseminated with washed sperm from her HIV-infected male partner. Even in states where people with HIV are allowed to donate, some fertility centers are unable to offer services to discordant couples. The laboratories require additional space and equipment to work with sperm samples from HIV-infected men and ensure that they are kept separate from other samples. Although an increasing number of fertility centers are offering sperm washing to discordant couples, it may be difficult to find such a center and couples may need to travel to use this service. Even fewer centers offer in vitro fertilization (IVF) with ICSI for decreasing the HIV transmission risk between partners.

If an HIV-infected woman becomes pregnant and does not receive any treatment, she has a greater than 1 in 5 (20%) chance of transmitting HIV to her baby. However, with appropriate obstetrical care, the risk declines to less than 1 percent. The key intervention to decrease HIV transmission risk from mother to child is drug therapy. The drugs that are recommended to decrease mother-to-fetus transmission have no major side effects for the baby. Some women may also be advised to deliver by Cesarean section.

Hepatitis

Since hepatitis B and C are transmitted in the same way as HIV, the strategies to decrease the risk of sexual transmission from partner to partner are similar to those for HIV. In addition to using insemination techniques, people with a hepatitis B or C infection should have their infection under control through medical treatments before they attempt conception. As in HIV infection, the status of the hepatitis infection can be monitored by checking the level of virus in the blood, and treatments can lower the hepatitis virus to undetectable levels.

Both hepatitis B and C can be transmitted from mother to child during pregnancy. Two or three of every 10 pregnant women with hepatitis B will transmit the infection to their child if they don't receive medical treatment. Fortunately, the available treatments are highly effective. The combined use of hepatitis B immune globulin and the hepatitis B vaccine protects 85 to 90 percent of babies from acquiring the infection from their mother. In other words, only about 1 in 10 women with hepatitis B who are treated with immune globulin and the vaccine will transmit the hepatitis B infection to their baby.

Pregnant women with hepatitis C have a 10 percent chance of transmitting the infection to their baby, unless they are also infected with HIV, in which case the risk increases. An HIV-positive woman with a large amount of hepatitis C virus in her blood has a 36 percent chance of transmitting the hepatitis C to her baby. Unfortunately, there is no treatment for hepatitis C that can be given during pregnancy to decrease the risk of transmitting the infection from mother to child. Women who are not pregnant and who are taking medication for hepatitis C treatment (interferon and ribavirin) should not become pregnant, because both of these drugs can potentially harm the fetus. However, women who have finished their course of hepatitis C treatment can become pregnant. If they have responded successfully to the treatment, their risk of transferring the infection to their baby may be greatly diminished.

FURTHER READING

COLAGE, Children of Lesbians and Gays Everywhere (an international organization that supports young people who have gay, lesbian, bisexual, and transgender parents). www.colage.org (415-861-KIDS).

National Adoption Center. www.adopt.org (215-735-9988 or 1-800-TO-ADOPT).

National Council for Single Adoptive Parents (an organization that can provide a listing of adoption agencies that will work with you to locate a foreign child or children). www.adopting.org/ncsap.html (ncsap@hotmail.com).

PACT: An Adoption Alliance (an organization that facilitates adoption for children of color). www.Pactadopt.org (415-221-6957).

SPAN, Single Parent Adoption Network. http://members.aol.com/onemomfor2.

I AM A FORTY-TWO-YEAR-OLD gay white man, and for many years I've wanted to raise children. I initially explored the idea of fathering a child with my previous partner and a lesbian couple who were friends of ours. We were unable to agree on the extent to which the four of us would be involved in parenting, so the plan didn't come to fruition. I then explored the idea of a lesbian friend acting as a surrogate. She would carry the child and at birth I would become the full-time parent. She would be acknowledged as the mother and would be involved peripherally with raising the child. She already had three adolescent children and they objected strongly, so the idea was dropped.

For the past four years, I have been in a relationship with a man of another ethnicity (African American). We are both interested in raising children and would like to adopt two children, preferably biracial or African American children. We would prefer to adopt one infant and one older child (three to seven years of age). Same-sex couples can't adopt a child together in the state we live in, so the plan is for me to apply to adoption agencies. After the adoption, we would work with a lawyer to make my partner a legal parent to the children, in case something happens to me.

We have also been discussing with my partner's family the possibility of adopting one of his cousin's children. His (male) cousin has several children and the mother of the youngest two was recently incarcerated, so the children are currently in foster care. The children's father hasn't decided what to do yet, but we hope that he will consider us as parents if he decides to give up the children.

My major regret is that I waited so long to begin the process. I wish I had started in my late twenties or early thirties. The thought of raising an adolescent when I am in my late fifties or early sixties is a bit intimidating.

PART II

Balancing the Risks and Benefits for Each Pathway

This section describes how you might balance the risks and benefits as you consider your options. How important is a genetic link and your influence on the fetal and infant environments? What are the medical and mental health risks of each option to your baby? What is the potential for emotional trauma (and corresponding highs)? How much will each pathway cost and how long will it take to become a parent? What are the legal issues you need to be concerned about?

Chapter 10

YOUR INFLUENCE ON GENETICS AND THE FETAL AND INFANT ENVIRONMENTS

For many people, the most compelling reason to choose a specific pathway to parenthood is the influence they can have on their child's genetic background and on the environment their child is exposed to from conception through early infancy. Numerous studies show that an adverse fetal environment or prolonged poor conditions early in a child's life can have long-term medical, emotional, cognitive, or developmental consequences.

Everyone feels different about how much influence they want to have on their child's genetic makeup, and only you can determine if this issue is a critical part of your decision. Of course, people who are unable to use their own eggs or sperm have less choice about how much genetic influence they can have. Many people would want to have as much involvement as possible in their child's early months and years of life, but again, opinions and feelings differ from person to person. This chapter reviews the degree of influence you can have on your child's genetic background and environment with fertility assistance, surrogacy, and adoption. We also describe environmental risks that you should know about as you weigh your options and make a decision about parenthood.

YOUR CHILD'S GENETIC BACKGROUND

For some people, a genetic link to their child is vital. For other people, a genetic link is not as important and they are willing to explore other options. In certain circumstances, it may not be possible to have a genetic link because of the potential for an inheritable disease. Maternal age is also a factor, because, as mentioned earlier in the book, a woman's age is correlated with chromosomal abnormalities. People considering the use of donor sperm, eggs, or embryos may be concerned about the donor's unknown genetic background. Checking the genetic background of a donor is an essential part of the donor screening process, however, so the possibility of a child inheriting a genetic problem from a donor is quite low.

Genetic Background When Using Your Own Eggs or Sperm

Of all the options for parenthood that we discuss in this book, the only one that allows you and your partner to have comprehensive knowledge about your child's genetic background is the use of your own eggs and sperm. If there is any question of an inheritable disease or a chromosome problem, you should be evaluated by an expert in genetics. A genetic evaluation usually involves a detailed family history and blood tests to screen for possible genetic defects. Below, we briefly describe the four major types of genetic defects: chromosomal abnormalities, polygenic defects, single-gene defects, and X-linked defects.

A chromosomal abnormality occurs when a child has the wrong number of chromosomes or an abnormal chromosome. For example, a child born with Down syndrome has an extra copy of one of the chromosomes (chromosome 21). A variety of syndromes occur as a result of a chromosomal abnormality. Depending on which chromosome is involved, the syndrome may be more or less severe. Some chromosome syndromes are so severe that the fetus is unable to develop and the pregnancy miscarries, whereas other syndromes allow a child to grow and lead a productive life into his or her adult years.

Polygenic defects result from a faulty interaction between two or more genes (segments of the DNA in a chromosome). Polygenic defects usually affect normal development of a specific organ. For example, polygenic defects associated with mouth development may result in a child being born with a cleft palate.

A single-gene disorder is caused by a defect in only one pair of genes. For every pair of genes, a child inherits one gene from the mother and one from the father. Every gene comes in one of two types, dominant or recessive, so a pair of genes may include two dominants, two recessives, or one dominant and one recessive. With a single-gene disorder, one of the two genes in the pair is defective, but whether or not the defect causes a problem in the person depends on the combination of dominant and recessive types.

With a dominant single-gene disorder, people who carry one faulty gene are somewhat affected by the disease, and those with two faulty genes can be more severely affected. For example, familial hypercholesterolemia is a dominant single-gene disorder characterized by very high cholesterol and premature heart disease. People with one faulty gene have a cholesterol level of around 400 mg/dl (a normal level is 200 mg/dl), and those with two faulty genes have cholesterol levels near 1,000 mg/dl. Other diseases caused by a single dominant gene include Huntington's disease and Marfan syndrome. A child conceived from an unaffected parent and an affected parent with one faulty gene has a 1 in 2 (or 50%) chance of inheriting the faulty gene from the affected parent and having the disorder. If the affected parent has two faulty genes, then the child will definitely get one of these genes and will have the disorder. If each parent has one faulty gene (which is highly unlikely), the child has a 1 in 4 chance of inheriting two faulty genes, a 1 in 2 chance of inheriting one faulty and one normal gene, and a 1 in 4 chance of inheriting two normal genes.

People with a disorder caused by a recessive gene, unlike those with a disease caused by a dominant gene, usually don't have symptoms of the disease and may not even realize they are carriers. But if two people who carry the recessive gene for a disorder have a child, their child has a 1 in 4 chance of receiving both recessive genes and being affected by the disorder. Some examples of recessive single-gene disorders are cystic fibrosis, Tay-Sachs disease, and thalassemia. Since they have no symptoms, the parents may have no idea that they carry the recessive gene until their child is born with the disease. Nearly 1,500 diseases are thought to be caused by dominant single-gene defects and about 1,100 by recessive single-gene defects.

The final type of genetic defect is an X-linked disorder. These disorders most often affect male children who inherit a faulty gene from their mother. Women have two X chromosomes, and a mother passes one of them to her child. If a woman carries a faulty gene on one of her X chromosomes, there is a 1 in 2 chance that her child will get the faulty gene. If the child is a girl, she also has an X chromosome from her father, and the normal gene on this X chromosome will override the faulty gene. She will not be affected by the disorder, but she (like her mother) will be a carrier. If the child is a boy, he has a Y chromosome from his father, so the faulty gene on the X chromosome is not overridden and the boy will have the disorder. A female child can only be affected by the disorder if her mother is a carrier, her father is affected by the disorder, and the child inherits the faulty gene on both X chromosomes. Two examples of X-linked disorders are color blindness and hemophilia.

Genetic Testing of a Fetus or Embryo

Once you conceive, you may decide to undergo a procedure that can detect genetic problems in the fetus. The three available procedures are chorionic villus sampling (CVS), amniocentesis, and preimplantation genetic diagnosis (PGD). CVS and amniocentesis are widely available, but PGD, which is done before the transfer of an embryo in an in vitro fertilization (IVF) cycle, is available only at some fertility centers.

CVS testing can be done as early as 10 weeks into a pregnancy. Depending on where the placenta is located, the chorionic villi (tissue cells in the placenta) can be sampled via a thin plastic tube inserted through the cervix or via a small needle inserted through the abdomen. With ultrasound guidance, the doctor pulls a small amount of tissue into a syringe. The test takes about five minutes and the discomfort is minimal (similar to a Pap smear). A repeat ultrasound is done two to four days after the test to be sure that everything looks fine. Complications can include infection, bleeding, and miscarriage. Fetal loss occurs in about 2 percent of procedures (a risk of 1 in 50).

Amniocentesis can be performed at 12 to 16 weeks gestation. Using ultrasound guidance, the doctor inserts a needle either through the mother's abdominal wall or through the vagina and then through the uterus to reach the amniotic sac. A small sample of amniotic fluid is obtained for testing. Although the procedure is routine, possible complications include infection, continued leakage of the fluid, and miscarriage. Fetal loss occurs in fewer than 1 percent of cases (the risk is between 1 in 1,600 and 1 in 200).

Neither CVS nor amniocentesis is 100 percent accurate. An abnormality may be present but not detected (a false negative), because some embryos have normal and abnormal cells and, by chance, only the normal cells may be sampled. If the results of a CVS or amniocentesis test show that a fetus is probably affected by a chromosomal abnormality or genetic disorder, the parents must decide whether they want to terminate the pregnancy. Sometimes the disorder is so severe that the fetus won't survive, and so the decision is perhaps a little easier. (And some couples choose to carry the fetus to term, knowing that the baby may die before birth or soon after birth.) In other cases, though, a fetus will survive and the child will live, albeit with medical problems.

PGD testing of an embryo created during an IVF procedure is usually done on day 3 of culture in the laboratory, when the embryo has four to nine cells. During the embryo biopsy, the outer layer (the zona pellucida) is opened by mechanical, chemical, or laser techniques and one or two cells are removed. Because PGD is a relatively new technique, there is limited information about any adverse effects on embryos. A large number of eggs need to be retrieved to do PGD testing, because not all eggs will be fertilized and progress to a stage at which a biopsy can be done. Most embryos (96%) survive the biopsy procedure, but pregnancy rates are slightly lower with biopsied embryos than with conventional IVF (16% for biopsied embryos versus 23% for nonbiopsied embryos, per treatment cycle).

Embryo biopsy with PGD testing can check for a variety of disorders. Disorders frequently screened for by PGD include cystic fibrosis, beta-thalassemia, sickle cell disease, spinal muscular atrophy, myotonic dystrophy, Huntington's disease, Charcot-Marie-Tooth disease, fragile X syndrome, hemophilia A, and Duchenne muscular dystrophy. As technology advances, it is possible that most genetic problems will be detectable. In one study, false negative results from PGD testing occurred in fewer than 1 percent of the births.

There are two main groups of people for whom PGD testing is indicated. The first group is couples at risk of transmitting a single-gene defect, an X-linked disorder, or another chromosomal abnormality. The second group is women who may have an increased chance of a chromosomal defect because of a history of recurrent miscarriages or repeated unsuccessful implantations. The test results can assist in determining which embryos should be transferred. The Ethics Committee of the American Society for Reproductive Medicine recommends that PGD be used solely for medical reasons, not for nonmedical reasons such as sex selection.

A recent study showed that using PGD in older women (ages thirty-five to forty-one years) to screen for an abnormal number of chromosomes did not result in a higher birth rate. In fact, for every nine women in this age group who planned to try three cycles of IVF or IVF plus ICSI, there was one less live birth when PGD testing was performed. The slightly lower birth rate with PGD probably occurred because the test reduced the pool of good-quality embryos from which to select for transfer to the uterus.

Given these results, PGD testing is not recommended solely because of older maternal age.

Genetic Background When Using
Donor Sperm, Eggs, or Embryos

If you decide to pursue the use of donor sperm, eggs, or embryos, you do have some choice regarding the genetic background. You can make reasonable requests of the donor program so that you are only presented with relatively compatible donors. Donor programs usually provide limited information on the donor's appearance (such as height, build, hair and eye color), ethnic origin, and family history, and they may include other characteristics such as educational background or personality. Ideally, they want to match recipients with a donor of the same race or races. They also perform very careful screening to minimize the risk of a child inheriting a genetic condition. If you plan to use a donor, request information from the agency or the fertility center about the extent of its donor screening process.

With the information recipients get, they can choose the donor they want to use. However, they may not have the luxury of being as selective for donor eggs or embryos as they can be for donor sperm. A wide selection of sperm donors is immediately available, regardless of whether the sperm are obtained from a sperm bank or a fertility center. But the same is not true for donor eggs or preexisting embryos, particularly at fertility centers. Eggs and embryos are always more difficult to get than sperm. If you are very selective, you are likely to have a relatively long wait for potential donor eggs or embryos. If you turn down an available donor, you may then wait several weeks or even months before having another donor option.

By searching on the internet to find a donor, you can be more selective. Several donor programs post extremely detailed portfolios on their donors. To get an idea of available donors, do an internet search for "sperm or egg or embryo donor."

As described in chapter 5, people interested in embryo adoption can be recipients of a preexisting embryo or can create embryos from donor eggs and sperm. Creating embryos offers more genetic options than adopting preexisting embryos, because the recipients decide which donors to use to create the embryo.

Genetic Background and Adoption

Adoptive parents have some influence over the genetic background of their child by choosing to adopt a child of a particular ethnicity. If you are very selective you will probably need to wait longer for a compatible infant or child, particularly if you use an agency and only want to adopt a healthy Caucasian baby. Conversely, if you are from a particular religious background and wish to adopt within your religion, you may have an easier time because some adoption agencies cater primarily to people of a specific religion.

In the case of international adoptions, it can be difficult to obtain medical information about the parents and other family members of a child available for adoption. The family genetic history is often not known, and a child may have a genetic condition that is not diagnosed as quickly as it otherwise might be or that becomes apparent only later in life.

THE FETAL, EARLY INFANT, AND EARLY CHILDHOOD ENVIRONMENTS

The fetal environment during the nine months of pregnancy has implications for the child's health and later development. People who decide to try fertility assistance and successfully conceive have the advantage of complete influence over the fetal environment. Those who pursue surrogacy or nonagency domestic adoptions may have some influence over the fetal environment, but ultimately the birth mother is in control. In most cases, prospective parents develop a relationship with the birth mother and know what kind of prenatal care she is receiving. If you financially support a birth mother, including paying her medical bills, you can be fairly comfortable that she is receiving appropriate nutrition and medical services. Nobody can prohibit a birth mother from participating in recreational activities, but regular contact usually allows prospective parents to have a good idea of whether she is drinking alcohol or using drugs. If a birth mother is using drugs or alcohol, and depending on the contractual agreement, the prospective parents may be able to choose whether or not to continue the relationship.

Open adoptions done through an agency also allow prospective parents to meet the birth mother, although they don't pay the bills directly and probably have less contact than in surrogacy or non-agency domestic adoptions. In closed private agency adoptions, there is no contact with the birth mother. Although the degree of influence over the fetal environment varies, if you choose to become a parent through surrogacy or by adopting an infant, you will have complete influence over the baby's environment very early in life.

Domestic public agency adoptions and international adoptions provide no opportunity for influence over the fetal environment and little chance of influence over the child's early life, because adopting a young infant is nearly impossible. It is more likely that the adopted child will be a toddler, so there may be no or only limited information about the pregnancy. It may not even be possible to find out if there were pregnancy complications or if the mother was using drugs or alcohol. The environment during a child's early infancy may not be well known either, including whether the child received adequate medical care and whether the child was neglected or abused. Frequently, children available for international adoption have been abandoned by their birth mother or birth parents, but generally there is no specific information about where or why the child was abandoned. Internationally adopted children from developing countries tend to have slightly higher rates of preadoption malnutrition, neglect, or abuse, but possibly fewer genetic problems, than their domestic peers.

Substance Use among Birth Mothers

The substances most commonly abused and known to have detrimental effects on the fetus are opiates (such as heroin), cocaine, alcohol, and nicotine. Each one of these substances can have adverse effects on the fetus and can cause problems prior to delivery and throughout a child's life.

How prevalent is such substance use by women who place their children for adoption? Should you be concerned about it? The National Adoption Information Clearinghouse (now part of the Child Welfare Information Gateway) gives the following statistics for the United States (or North America):

- Every year, 2.6 million infants are exposed to alcohol during the mother's pregnancy.
- Every year, fetal alcohol syndrome (FAS) affects between 1.3 and 2.2 babies per 1,000 live births in North America.
- Cases of babies with fetal alcohol effects (FAE) outnumber cases of babies with FAS.*
- Every year, 11 percent of all newborns—more than 450,000 babies—are exposed to illicit drugs during the pregnancy.
- Every year, more than 739,000 women use one or more illicit drugs during pregnancy.
- The rate of birth of substance-exposed infants exceeds one birth every 90 seconds.

Mothers who have an addiction are often not able to take care of their children and are at risk for having their children placed in foster care. Many of these children later become available for adoption.

Substance use is not confined to birth mothers of children adopted domestically. Exposure to alcohol is also a problem for infants adopted from several other countries, particularly some countries in Eastern Europe and the former Soviet Union. For ex-

---

* A fetus can suffer a variety of problems due to exposure to alcohol. The term fetal alcohol syndrome was introduced in 1973 and is defined by specific diagnostic criteria, including certain facial abnormalities, growth retardation, and neurodevelopmental abnormalities of the central nervous system. However, some babies are adversely affected by prenatal alcohol exposure but do not meet the criteria for FAS. These babies are described as having fetal alcohol effects. Babies with FAE but not FAS may have one or more congenital, central nervous system, behavioral, or cognitive defects or deficits.

ample, Richard Barth and coauthors, in a chapter in the book *Adoption and Prenatal Alcohol and Drug Exposure*, estimate that the rate of FAS in the former Soviet Union is potentially eight times greater than the worldwide incidence. The potential consequences for a fetus and child of exposure to alcohol or drugs are described in chapter 12.

The Environment for Infants and Toddlers

If you decide to adopt either domestically with a public agency or internationally, you need to be concerned about the quality of your child's environment when he or she was an infant and toddler. The time between birth and 18 months is critical for a child's emotional and cognitive development. The parent-child relationship influences all of a child's future relationships. By 18 months, children with secure attachments to nurturing parents believe that their parents will come back after brief absences and that their parents will meet their needs by providing consistent care, comfort, soothing, and attention. Babies and young children learn when and how to appropriately signal for help—with behaviors like crying or clinging—when they become frustrated or frightened or are in pain. Unfortunately, children without reliable parents during their first year of life do not learn how to develop a trusting relationship. Early maternal separation and deprivation can have serious developmental consequences for infants and older children and they may have difficulty with future relationships.

Children who do not have parents who respond to their needs may fail to thrive, have problems with motor coordination, appear confused or unfocused, lack joyful responses, avoid eye contact, and fuss when held. They often won't approach other people and don't develop usual responses to social interactions. Equally concerning are children who are excessively familiar or uninhibited with other people. These children may cling to complete strangers rather than to their parent or parents, and they may look to strangers for comfort or affection. Situations that can interrupt parent-child attachment include orphanage care, parents with drug or alcohol addiction, parents with major depression and other mental health conditions, and traumas to a child such as sexual abuse, physical abuse, domestic violence, and neglect. The effects of insecure attachments are discussed further in chapter 12.

The Environment for International Infants

Although some countries place children awaiting adoption into foster homes, most children awaiting international adoption live in orphanages where the conditions may not be optimal. Many orphanages are understaffed and lack other resources. Children living in these orphanages often suffer from emotional and social deprivation as well as some degree of nutritional deprivation, although the malnutrition is usually mild to moderate. Children with severe nutritional deprivation usually are not selected for adoption. Some countries have made huge strides in the past few years toward improving the quality of orphanage care. Potential consequences of malnutrition are outlined in chapter 11. Table 10.1 summarizes the preadoption living situation and ages of children available for adoption from selected foreign countries.

If you decide to adopt internationally, you can use several strategies to smooth the transition to life together in the United States for you and your child or children. The following tips will help you know what to expect:

- Consider counseling before you receive your child to help you prepare for the emotional and behavioral challenges you may face in the near future.
- Investigate your child's culture of origin to learn about practices such as holding, bathing, feeding, sleeping, dressing, diapering, and toileting. If possible, visit the orphanage, baby home, or foster home where your child has been living to learn more about its care-giving procedures. Your ideas about child care may be quite different from the care your child is used

Table 10.1. The Preadoption Setting and Age of Children in Ten Countries

Country	Setting	Age of child
China	Orphanage	Infants to 6 years; older and special needs children
Russia[1]	Orphanage	>10 months
Guatemala	Orphanage or foster care	Infants; young children; older and special needs children
South Korea	Foster care and group homes	>6 months
Ukraine[2]	Orphanage	Toddlers >15 months; older and special needs children
Kazakhstan	Orphanage	Infants; toddlers; older and special needs children
Ethiopia	Orphanage or foster care	Infants; toddlers; older children
India	Orphanage	Infants; young children; special needs children
Colombia	Orphanage	Newborn to 18 months
Philippines	Orphanage or foster care	6 months to 10 years; special needs children

Source: U.S. State Department. Country Specific Information about Adoption (www.travel
.state.gov/family/adoption/country_369.html).

1. Videotape of child is usually available after referral is made.

2. Unlike other countries, Ukraine does not disclose information on children available for
adoption to agencies or other private citizens. Adoptive parents who have registered with the
State Department for Adoptions and Protection of Rights of the Child (SDAPRC) may
receive information about available children only after they have received an invitation from
SDAPRC to travel to Ukraine.

to receiving, and easing your child into your routines will result
in less stress for you and your new child.

- Become well informed about the cultural values and characteristics of your child's birth country. Having this information will assist you in supporting your child when he or she
is older and struggles with his or her identity. This knowledge will also equip you in helping your child overcome racial
or ethnic challenges at school or in the community.

- After you and your child have had a chance to settle into a routine, obtain a full, multidisciplinary developmental assessment (pediatric, psychological, etc.). Depending on the age of the child, bilingual clinicians may be needed. This early evaluation can help to identify any social, emotional, developmental, and medical concerns so that appropriate therapy or other interventions can begin.

POSITIVE ASPECTS TO CONSIDER

- With fertility assistance options, you have influence over your child's genetic background.
- Medical advances, such as PGD, have made it possible to select embryos that are not affected by specific genetic disorders.
- If you carry a pregnancy, you have complete control over the fetal environment.
- With surrogacy and some adoptions, you can choose to be highly involved in the pregnancy so that you know about the fetal environment.
- Depending on the type of adoption, you can decide to stop pursuing the adoption of a particular child if you have concerns about the fetal environment or the child's early life.
- By adopting an infant, you will have complete control over the child's early life. By adopting an older child, you will have an opportunity to make a difference in that child's life.

FURTHER READING

L. B. Andrews. *New Conceptions: A Consumer's Guide to the Newest Infertility Treatments.* Ballantine Books, 1985.

D. D. Gray. *Attaching in Adoption.* Perspectives Press, 2002.

R. Mintzer. *Yes, You Can Adopt! A Comprehensive Guide to Adoption.* Avalon, Carroll and Graf, 2003.

National Adoption Information Clearinghouse. Adoption Statistics: Drug Exposure. Available at: http://statistics.adoption.com/drug_exposed_infants.php.

MY HUSBAND AND I HAD MANY YEARS to consider different pathways to parenthood. I have uterine problems, so I knew early on in our marriage that I couldn't physically carry my own child. My ovaries, however, were fine. The options available to us were gestational surrogacy, traditional surrogacy, and adoption.

We were both in our early thirties when the time came to start our family. We considered all the options carefully. We liked the idea of adopting, but we also liked the idea of having our own genetic child. We would have qualified for both domestic and international adoption, but we were concerned with the prenatal and the immediate postnatal environments. Even with surrogacy, we knew that we must deal with prenatal control issues, but at the time it seemed to us that we could have better control with surrogacy than with adoption. We decided to try gestational surrogacy, given that out of all options it would offer us the most control (particularly the ability to have genetic control). We decided up-front to try only three IVF attempts, surrogate willing, and if these should fail we would move on to international or domestic adoption.

Thankfully, we have had an amazingly good experience with gestational surrogacy. We found an ideal match and have built a wonderful friendship with our carrier. Our carrier doesn't live near us, but travel and coordination of monitoring through the preconception and postconception process have been very smooth—probably due to experienced clinics and also to a large and experienced surrogacy agency. The first IVF attempt failed, but the second attempt was successful. In both attempts we implanted only two fresh, day 5 embryos (blastocysts). In the second attempt, both embryos implanted and one divided! At the time of writing, we are in week 16 of our pregnancy and are expecting triplets—two of whom will be identical. We are thrilled, excited, and nervous.

Our surrogate wanted so badly to give someone the chance of parenthood and now she's giving it to us. We are very involved with her and the pregnancy and attend most prenatal visits. Our surrogate has a very supportive husband and three young children. She has been open and honest with her children, just as my husband and I plan to be with our children. We'll tell them about their conception as soon as possible, but we also understand that it may not be as easy as we think.

It's been nearly a year since we first signed on with an agency, and we're still amazed at all that has happened. The only thing we might have done differently would be to think more fully about the IVF process and the chance of a high-risk, multiple pregnancy. We didn't think the chance of embryo division was very high. However, at this time, our triplets are doing fine. Despite the risks involved in a higher-order pregnancy, the chance of being parents to not one but three children of our own is something we never dreamed possible.

Chapter 11

PREGNANCY AND MEDICAL RISKS FOR MOTHER AND CHILD

No matter which pathway you choose to become a parent, there will be medical risks. No one option can guarantee a safe pregnancy and a healthy child. Of course, medical problems for the mother and child or children are not inevitable. Many pregnancies, surrogacies, and adoptions progress with no or few problems, and the end result is a healthy mother, happy parents, and a thriving child. Nevertheless, you should be aware of the risks, so in this chapter we discuss the most common obstetrical (pregnancy) complications for the birth mother and the most common medical disorders for the child or children.

RISKS FROM FERTILITY ASSISTANCE PROCEDURES

Rarely do serious complications occur with the minimally invasive procedures involved in the initial fertility workup. As described in chapter 1, short-term mild to moderate discomfort or pain is usual following some of the procedures.

The fertility assistance procedures themselves carry some risks. Some women are especially prone to adverse side effects from the hormones used in fertility interventions. As described in chapter 2, common side effects include headache, bloating, weight gain, and mood swings. A more serious complication, which occurs in about 3 of every 100 women who undergo an assisted reproductive technology (ART) cycle, is ovarian hyperstimulation syndrome (OHSS). OHSS occurs when a woman's body responds too well to the hormone stimulation and her estrogen rises to tremendously high levels. This complication can be dangerous and potentially fatal. The estimated mortality rate is 1 per 450,000 to 500,000 cases of OHSS. Symptoms include difficulty urinating, difficulty breathing, and sudden weight gain of 10 pounds or more in less than a week (for example, a woman may gain more than 2 pounds a day following the injections). Other disorders, including infections or blood clots, can be associated with OHSS.

Two types of OHSS can occur. One, an early-onset pattern, occurs within the first nine days after the eggs are retrieved. In this case, the syndrome is probably due to one or both ovaries overresponding to the hormone stimulation. The ovaries continue to mature follicles and they also produce too much estrogen. The second type, a late-onset pattern, occurs on or after day 10 following egg retrieval and is thought to be caused by a pregnancy hormone, beta human chorionic gonadotropin (hCG), which is produced when an embryo implants. Late-onset OHSS tends to be more severe.

When a woman begins a hormone stimulation cycle, she is monitored closely to ensure that follicle development and estrogen increases are controlled. If too many follicles develop during a hormone stimulation cycle, or if the estrogen levels are too high, the fertility specialist should consider canceling the cycle. If a cycle is canceled and the hormone injections are stopped, the estrogen level drops quickly. A woman who develops mild symptoms of OHSS will be advised by her physician to drink clear liquids and limit her activities. Women who have severe symptoms may need to be admitted into the hospital and undergo more aggressive measures, such as draining excess fluid from the abdominal cavity and administration of intravenous albumin (a type of protein). Pregnancy can prolong the symptoms of OHSS; it may take up to 10 weeks for the symptoms to disappear (resolve) in a pregnant woman. A woman who has been treated for OHSS can try hormone stimulation treatment again, but the hormone regimen will need to be individualized using lower doses and the woman must be carefully monitored.

Another rare complication, which occurs in fewer than 1 in 100 women, is twisting of the ovary. This condition needs to be surgically repaired. If the twisting, referred to as ovarian torsion, is diagnosed and treated early, the ovary will most likely remain functional. However, if treatment is delayed, the blood supply to the ovary is cut off, which results in tissue death and compromises the woman's fertility. ART procedures may also cause infections, though infrequently. There are other fertility interventions that a physician may recommend trying in particular cases, and these interventions will have specific risks. If a physician suggests that you undergo another procedure, ask about the risks.

Many women worry about the possibility of cancer after taking high doses of hormones, but there is little evidence to support this concern.

RISKS DURING PREGNANCY

Many women want very much to be pregnant and they enjoy their pregnancy. For others, however, pregnancy is an uncomfortable condition, particularly when carrying multiples. A variety of complications can occur during pregnancy and, as outlined in table 11.1, the risk for many of them increases with maternal age and for women who become pregnant with ART.

Certain pregnancy complications are associated with age, particularly if the mother is over forty years old. Pregnancy-related hypertension has been reported in as many as 1 in 3 women age fifty years or older (who become pregnant through donor eggs because of their age). Diabetes occurring during pregnancy is another relatively common condition and occurs in approximately 6 to 17 percent of pregnant women over forty years of age. Fetal mortality nearly doubles among mothers age forty years and older compared with mothers younger than thirty. This difference is primarily seen among mothers who are carrying just one child.

Table 11.1. Obstetrical Complications Related to Maternal Age or Assisted Reproductive Technology (ART)

Complication	Increased risk with maternal age	Increased risk with ART
Pregnancy-induced hypertension	Yes	Yes
Premature delivery	Yes	Yes
Low-birth-weight infant	Yes	Yes
Miscarriage and stillbirth	Yes	Yes
Diabetes	Yes	Yes
Cardiac disease	Yes	No
Abruptio placentae[1]	Yes	Yes
Placenta previa[2]	Yes	Yes
Ectopic pregnancy[3]	Yes	Yes
Anemia	No	Yes
Excess amniotic fluid	Yes	Yes
Cesarean section	Yes	Yes
Excessively large birth weight	Yes	No

1. In abruptio placentae, the placenta separates early from the uterus, causing bleeding and possible fetal complications or death.

2. In placenta previa, the placenta completely or partially covers the opening of the uterus and can cause bleeding during the second or third trimesters.

3. An ectopic pregnancy occurs in the fallopian tubes. The embryo cannot survive, and the woman may lose function of the tube.

On the other hand, maternal age does not seem to affect the risk of adverse birth outcomes—such as miscarriage, stillbirth, and birth defects—among mothers giving birth to multiples, unless the mother is over fifty years of age.

Women who have become pregnant with ART also seem to be at greater risk of other complications, such as very high blood pressure at time of delivery (a condition known as preeclampsia), placental problems, Cesarean section, and premature deliveries. Pregnancies achieved by hormone stimulation and intrauterine insemination (IUI) are also at higher risk for these complications. It is unclear whether these increased risks are attributable to underlying infertility, characteristics of the infertile couple, or ART.

Risks in a Pregnancy with Multiples

As we have described, several fertility assistance methods use hormones to stimulate the woman's body to develop more than one mature egg. This induced multiple ovulation increases the risk of becoming pregnant with multiple fetuses. Twin pregnancies occur in 1 to 2 percent of women who become pregnant without fertility assistance. In women who take Clomid (described in chapter 2), the rate of twin pregnancies increases to 5 to 10 percent. Triplet and higher-order multiple pregnancies are rare with Clomid. When pregnancy occurs using hormone stimulation (injected hormones) in combination with either intercourse or insemination, 15 to 20 percent are twin gestations and 5 percent are triplets or higher-order multiples.

Pregnancies with multiples also occur in women undergoing ART procedures, because frequently more than one embryo is transferred into the uterus. The chance of pregnancy must be balanced against the risks of a high-order multiple pregnancy. Couples can lessen the chance of having multiples by transferring fewer embryos, but this strategy may also decrease the chances for conception. As shown in table 11.2, maternal age influences the chance of conception with ART, and so age is one of the primary

Table 11.2. Live Births and Multiple Pregnancy Rates for Women Using Their Own Eggs in Assisted Reproductive Technology Procedures

Maternal age in years	Percentage of cycles resulting in live births	Percentage of pregnancies with twins	Percentage of pregnancies with triplets or more
<35	36.9	32.7	5.1
35–37	29.3	28.0	5.6
38–40	19.5	21.2	4.4
41–42	10.7	14.5	2.5

Source: Society for Assisted Reproductive Technology data. Centers for Disease Control and Prevention. 2004 Assisted Reproductive Technology (ART) Report: National Summary (http://apps.nccd.cdc.gov/ART2004/nation04.asp).

Table 11.3. Recommended Number of Embryos to Transfer According
to Maternal Age

Maternal age in years[1]	Number of embryos[2]
<35	1–2
35–37	2–3
38–40	3–4
>40	≤5

Source: Adapted from Practice Committee of the Society for Assisted Reproductive Technology, Practice Committee of the American Society for Reproductive Medicine. Guidelines on
number of embryos transferred. *Fertil Steril* 2006;86(5 suppl):S51–52.

1. For donor eggs, age refers to the donor, not the recipient.

2. Factors that can affect the decision about how many embryos to transfer include
embryo quality, previous failure of in vitro fertilization (IVF), the IVF clinic's success rate,
and the couple's feelings about multiple births and selective reduction (fetal termination).

factors taken into account when determining how many embryos
to transfer. The Society for Assisted Reproductive Technology
(SART) and the American Society for Reproductive Medicine
(ASRM) provide guidelines on the recommended number of embryos to transfer according to a woman's age (table 11.3).

Most people who are trying to become parents have mixed feelings about a multiple pregnancy. On the one hand, they desperately want children, and giving birth to multiples means that they
immediately have a large family. On the other hand, having multiples, particularly three or more, dramatically increases complications during the pregnancy and potential problems for the health
of the babies. Both maternal and fetal complications are more
severe with a higher number of fetuses.

Pregnancy complications (see table 11.1) that are specifically
associated with multiple births include an increased risk of miscarriage, diabetes, pregnancy-induced hypertension, vaginal or
uterine bleeding, prolonged bed rest, and Cesarean section. Pregnancy loss rates before 24 weeks gestation are approximately 1 in
16 to 1 in 20 (5% to 6%) for twins and 1 in 8 to 1 in 9 (11% to
13%) for triplets.

Complications for the children of a multiple pregnancy include
an increased chance of preterm birth, birth defects, and lifelong

mental or physical handicaps. The vast majority of complications and medical problems experienced by these children occur because many women carrying multiples deliver too early. The normal length of gestation is 39 weeks. The average gestation is reduced to 35 weeks for twins, 33 weeks for triplets, and just 29 weeks for quadruplets. In general, the risk of complications from premature delivery is much less once the pregnancy reaches 32 to 34 weeks gestation. Physicians often put women carrying multiples on bed rest in an effort to increase the length of the gestation. A woman can expect at least one month of bed rest with twins and even longer for higher-order multiples.

Infant death rates also increase for babies from a multiple pregnancy. Compared with a singleton, a child born from a twin gestation is 4 times more likely to die in the first year of life, and a triplet is 10 times more likely to die. The chances of cerebral palsy also increase with multiples; for every 1,000 surviving infants, approximately 2 singletons, 7 to 12 twins, and 28 to 45 triplets have cerebral palsy. Some other studies have shown that triplets have up to a 1 in 3 risk of neurodevelopmental abnormalities, such as cognitive impairment or abnormal neuromuscular development including weakness or paralysis. The risk of complications is associated with gestational age. Triplets and higher-order multiples are at highest risk because they are more likely to be born before 32 weeks gestation.

Selective Reduction

When a woman becomes pregnant with multiples, she and her partner may want to consider a selective reduction (also called pregnancy reduction or selective termination). This option is also open to women carrying a surrogate pregnancy. The goal of a selective reduction is to abort one or more of the fetuses to give the remaining fetuses a better chance of developing and being born without complications and future health problems. Selective reduction is an outpatient procedure in which a physician inserts a needle through the woman's abdomen into the sac surrounding the fetus and injects a chemical solution, resulting in the death of the fetus. The woman's body subsequently absorbs the nonviable fetus and she never delivers any tissue. The procedure is most often done very early in pregnancy, at 9 to 12 weeks in the first trimester, but it can be performed as late as 24 weeks gestation. The risk of losing the remaining fetuses is approximately 1 in 10 to 1 in 20, but the overall risks for the pregnancy and health outcomes are lowered by the reduction procedure. About 3 of every 4 women who undergo a selective reduction have a premature labor later in the pregnancy. Infections in the mother are rare.

The issue of selective reduction should be discussed with the fertility specialist prior to beginning an ART procedure, so that the woman or couple will have decided what to do in the case of a multiple pregnancy. Their decision will also influence the number of embryos transferred. Regardless, it can still be difficult to decide to proceed with a reduction, and some people may need additional counseling. Unfortunately, the decision can't be delayed, particularly if a woman needs to travel out of her home state for the procedure. Not all fertility centers offer selective reduction services, so women who want to undergo the procedure may need to travel elsewhere.

UNPLANNED EVENTS

Miscarriage

In general, having a miscarriage is not a medically dangerous complication for a woman. The biggest toll of a miscarriage is emotional (see chapter 13). Many miscarriages occur because something is seriously wrong with the unborn child. Sixty percent or more of early miscarriages (miscarriages in the first trimester) may be caused by chromosomal abnormalities. As women age, they have a higher risk of carrying a fetus with a chromosomal abnormality, and so the miscarriage rate is also higher. A woman who becomes pregnant with her own eggs after age forty has a 1 in 66 (1.5%) chance of a chromosomal abnormality, and for a woman older than forty-five the risk increases to 1 in 21 (4.8%).

For women using their own eggs in an ART procedure, the miscarriage rate is 15 percent (1 in 6.7) among women younger than thirty-five years, 30 percent (1 in 3.3) at age forty, 41 percent (1 in 2.4) at age forty-three, and over 50 percent after age forty-five. Fortunately, fewer than 5 percent of women have two consecutive miscarriages and only 1 percent have three or more. About 1 in 20 couples have an inherited genetic cause of a chromosomal defect that leads to miscarriage. Couples with specific chromosomal defects may benefit from preimplantation genetic diagnosis (PGD) in conjunction with ART, as described in chapter 10.

Chromosomal Abnormalities

Physicians usually offer women over thirty-five years of age an elective amniocentesis because of the higher risk of chromosomal abnormalities. An amniocentesis is a routine outpatient procedure with little chance of complications, although 0.5 to 1 percent of women who have an amniocentesis subsequently miscarry. Amniocentesis is described in more detail in chapter 10.

Chromosomal abnormalities in a child are not always the result of a problem with the chromosomes in the mother's egg; abnormalities can also occur because of a problem with the sperm. Among infertile couples, about half of the male partners are found to have abnormal sperm. Infertile men with chromosomal abnormalities are more likely to have genetically abnormal sperm and to father chromosomally abnormal children. The proportion of men with either low sperm counts or no measurable sperm in the semen who have children with chromosomal abnormalities is 1 in 22 (4.6%) and 1 in 7 (13.7%), respectively. Some men without measurable sperm in their semen may still create sperm, but the sperm are not mixed with the rest of the ejaculatory fluid due to a physical obstruction. Other men without measurable sperm are born lacking the vas deferens (a muscular tube that connects the epididymis, where sperm are made, to the ejaculatory ducts). About two-thirds of men without the vas deferens have a genetic mutation that can cause cystic fibrosis if they conceive with a woman who also carries a gene for this condition (a recessive single-gene disorder, as explained in chapter 10).

Since 2000, the World Health Organization has recommended routine genetic screening for men with sperm levels of less than 5 million/ml of semen. Men with very low sperm counts should be offered counseling and testing for chromosomal abnormalities in their sperm before attempting IVF and intracytoplasmic sperm injection (ICSI). Depending on the results of sperm testing, they may wish to consider using a sperm donor. Men who have a structural defect preventing sperm from mixing with the ejaculate may benefit from surgical correction. Fertility specialists can also obtain sperm directly from the male reproductive system for the IVF procedure.

The chance of a chromosomal abnormality occurring in a fetus conceived by a couple in the general population (that is, without fertility assistance) is 2 in 1,000. After accounting for a woman's age and the number of children she already has, the use of standard IVF procedures has a 7 in 1,000 chance of producing a fetus with a chromosomal abnormality. This rate is not considered to be significantly different from that for the general population. In other words, IVF alone does not increase the risk of chromosomal abnormalities. However, couples who need to use ICSI because of a sperm problem do have a higher likelihood of having a child with a chromosome disorder when compared with the general population. Ten in 1,000 babies conceived with IVF plus ICSI have chromosomal abnormalities, and this higher rate may be due to the increased risk of chromosomal abnormalities for men with sperm problems.

Birth Defects

Studies have tried to evaluate whether babies conceived with ART have higher rates of major congenital malformations (birth defects). Congenital malformations can involve many different organs, such as the brain, heart, lungs, liver, bones, or gastrointestinal tract. Examples of congenital malformations include heart defects, cleft lip or palate, spina bifida, and limb defects. The results for the effects of ART are conflicting. Several studies find that approximately 2 percent of all babies have birth defects, regardless of whether they are conceived with ART or not (that is, in the general population). Other studies report that 5 to 9 percent of babies conceived with ART have birth defects.

One specific disorder that may occur more frequently in babies conceived through IVF plus ICSI is hypospadias. Hypospadias is a condition in males in which the opening of the urethra (where the urine comes out of the body) is on the underside of the penis. Mild cases of hypospadias are primarily a cosmetic defect, although the direction of the urinary stream is affected. More severe cases make urination messy and may require sitting to urinate. The man's fertility can also be affected. Hypospadias is treated surgically, with severe cases sometimes requiring several surgeries and skin grafting. Additional studies are ongoing to evaluate if hypospadias truly is more common among babies conceived by IVF plus ICSI.

The IVF procedure itself doesn't appear to have any significant adverse effects on an infant or child. The process of freezing embryos and then thawing them for transfer into the uterus also seems to have no negative effects.

Stillbirth

Stillbirth is the death of a fetus that has reached at least 20 weeks gestation. As with miscarriages, maternal age significantly increases the risk of a pregnancy ending in stillbirth. Data from the National Center for Health Statistics collected between 1997 and 1999 showed that the rates for stillbirth in the general population increased from 4 per 1,000 pregnancies for women between twenty and twenty-nine years of age to 10 per 1,000 for women older than forty years. Even though stillbirths are relatively rare, they are about 10 times as common as sudden infant death syndrome in babies born to older women. Although older women using donor eggs have a higher risk of selected obstetrical complications, they don't have the relatively high rates of miscarriage or stillbirth seen among women over forty years old who use their own eggs.

Postpartum Depression

Right after giving birth, the majority of women feel a mild moodiness or sadness that quickly goes away. These feelings are sometimes referred to as baby blues. More severe depression, called postpartum depression, is less common. The chances of a mother experiencing postpartum depression are 1 in 4 to 1 in 20 (5% to 25%). Using fertility assistance has not been shown to be a risk for postpartum depression, but because this can be a complication of any pregnancy, we describe it briefly. Symptoms can occur any time in the first year postpartum and include feelings of sadness, hopelessness, emptiness, and guilt; low self-esteem; sleeping and eating disturbances; low energy and exhaustion; an inability to be comforted or to enjoy activities previously enjoyed; social withdrawal; being easily frustrated; and feeling inadequate in taking care of the baby. A woman has a higher risk for postpartum depression if she has previously suffered depression, has little support, and the pregnancy was unplanned. The dramatic changes in hormone levels with pregnancy and childbirth may bring about the symptoms in some women but are not thought to be the main cause of postpartum depression for most women.

FETAL EXPOSURE TO HARMFUL SUBSTANCES

Children adopted domestically or internationally may have been affected by fetal drug, alcohol, or nicotine exposure. The primary drugs of concern are opiates, cocaine, and alcohol, because of the harmful effects these substances can have on the fetus.

Heroin and Other Opioid/Narcotic Drugs

- The fetus becomes physically dependent on the drug and suffers withdrawal symptoms after birth.

Cocaine/Crack

- Cocaine-exposed fetuses have a higher risk of premature birth, growth retardation, microcephaly (small head size), and abnormal brain development.
- Cocaine can slow or temporarily stop blood flow to the fetal brain, resulting in brain damage.

Alcohol

- Fetal alcohol exposure can cause fetal alcohol effects (FAE), fetal alcohol syndrome (FAS), or alcohol-related neurodevelopmental disorder (ARND).
- Babies with FAS can have slower growth, smaller heads, heart problems, facial abnormalities, developmental abnormalities of the central nervous system (including mental retardation), and a pattern of cognitive and behavioral abnormalities not explained by other factors.
- Babies with ARND are easily stressed and can have difficulty establishing sleeping patterns, toilet training, and personal space.

Nicotine

- Carbon monoxide from smoking causes intrauterine growth retardation, and nicotine causes brain cell damage.
- Women who smoke during pregnancy have more miscarriages, increased premature delivery rates, and babies with lower birth weights than women who do not smoke.
- A possible link has been identified between a woman smoking during pregnancy and her child having an attention deficit disorder (ADD) or other disturbances of the nervous system such as learning difficulties.
- Infants born to smokers are more jittery and excitable and are harder to console than the newborns of nonsmokers.

CHILDHOOD DEVELOPMENTAL PROBLEMS

Most children in orphanages display evidence of malnutrition and growth development problems. Generally, children are expected to lose about one month of linear growth (that is, growth in length or height) for every three months they spend in institutional care. Children in orphanages may also have slower brain growth. Although most children have dramatic catch-up growth after adoption, it is not yet known whether the recovery of brain mass means that the brain will function normally. Developmental delays are common in areas such as expressive language and gross and fine motor skills. Fortunately, the limited information we have shows that good nutrition at a young age combined with an improved psychosocial environment can ameliorate or even erase the developmental and growth delays due to early malnutrition. Unfortunately, children with prolonged social and nutritional deprivation have a poorer chance of complete recovery.

Doctors in the United States who specialize in evaluating children from other countries can screen for major disorders by watching videotapes of a child. However, detecting mild to moderate developmental delay by video review is challenging. If videotapes are not available, some doctors will also use photographs to assess a child, although there are obvious limitations to how much they can determine. If it's difficult to obtain a photograph before you travel to the child's country, once in the country you could try sending photos or videos via the internet to obtain a professional opinion. Additional information on mental health disorders is given in chapter 12.

MEDICAL CONCERNS UNIQUE
TO INTERNATIONAL ADOPTION

Children adopted internationally often have several of the medical conditions already described, in addition to a variety of other conditions, which are listed in table 11.4. Most of these conditions are easily managed and do not have serious long-term effects. The most common infectious diseases are related to parasites and can be treated and cured. A few conditions, namely congenital syphilis, HIV, and hepatitis B and C, can have serious consequences. One in 10 to 1 in 20 Asian children and 1 in 5 Romanian children have chronic hepatitis B. HIV infection is not included in table 11.4, but it can occur. In Ethiopia, for example, if a child has two parents with HIV/AIDS, the government routinely declares the child to be an orphan. These children, some of whom have HIV, may be eligible for adoption. Most children in

Table 11.4. Medical Conditions in Internationally Adopted Children

Conditions commonly reported by the country
- Family history of mental illness or mental retardation
- Drug or alcohol exposure before birth
- Prematurity
- Low birth weight
- History of abuse/neglect
- Prolonged or recurrent hospitalization/institutionalization
- Malnutrition
- Rickets
- Anemia[1]
- Recurrent respiratory infections
- Incomplete immunization
- Hepatitis B and C[2]
- Syphilis in the mother[3]
- Developmental dysplasia of the hip
- Developmental delay
- Decreased muscle tone

Conditions commonly confirmed or discovered after placement
- Growth deficiency
- Small head/brain
- Fetal alcohol syndrome
- Sexual or physical abuse (especially in older children)

(continued)

Table 11.4 *(continued)*

- Hepatitis B and C[2]
- Positive skin test for tuberculosis[4]
- Intestinal parasites[5]
- Scabies[6]
- Lead exposure[1]
- Cavities
- Strabismus (misaligned eyes)
- Developmental delay (especially speech and language)
- Behavioral problems
- Sleep disturbances
- Feeding difficulties
- Self-stimulating behaviors (for example, head banging)

Source: Adapted from J. M. Beidso and B. D. Johnston. Preparing families for international adoption. *Pediatr Rev* 2004;25:245.

1. Anemia is usually due to iron deficiency, other underlying medical conditions, or lead poisoning.

2. Chronic hepatitis B infection is highly prevalent in many countries where internationally adopted children originate. Between 2 and 20 percent of children have active hepatitis B that may need treatment. Hepatitis C infection is rare.

3. Congenital syphilis is identified rarely, but when it is, the child has been born with syphilis that causes problems such as an enlarged liver or spleen, a rash, or birth defects.

4. The chance of a tuberculosis infection in internationally adopted children is at least four to six times higher than for children born in the United States.

5. Gastrointestinal parasites that cause disease have been found in 9 to 51 percent of internationally adopted children. *Giardia lamblia* (giardia) is the most commonly identified parasite, and the highest frequency has been noted in children from Romania, Bulgaria, Moldova, Russia, and China.

6. Scabies, lice, and ringworm occur frequently.

international adoptions, except those from China, arrive with documentation of an HIV test done in their birth country.

It is not uncommon for doctors in a foreign country to note in a child's chart what they perceive as a significant medical problem. Many U.S. physicians are not familiar with the stated diagnoses, but fortunately, the problems are usually quite minor. Although not a medical problem, the exact birth date of some children is unknown and their age has to be estimated.

POSITIVE ASPECTS TO CONSIDER

- If you are over thirty-five years of age, using donor eggs can reduce the risk of chromosomal abnormalities.
- If you become pregnant with multiples, you will have an instant large family.
- If you use a surrogate or adopt, you won't need to worry about going through any pregnancy discomfort or experiencing complications yourself.
- Most medical conditions in internationally adopted children are easily managed and do not have long-term consequences.

FURTHER READING

D. D. Gray. *Attaching in Adoption.* Perspectives Press, 2002.
J. Meyers-Thompson and S. Perkins. *Fertility for Dummies.* Wiley, 2003.

MY HUSBAND AND I WENT THROUGH YEARS of fertility assistance, including several IVF attempts, without success. With every attempt, the stakes became higher. It seemed almost unbearable to stop trying, but could we afford to keep going? Given this dilemma, we chose to transfer more than two embryos at a time, knowing there was the possibility of a multiple gestation. We discussed the possibility of a fetal termination with our fertility specialist, if we were so lucky as to become pregnant with more than two babies.

On our fourth IVF attempt, we became pregnant with triplets. Even though we had thought about the possibility beforehand and had decided we would proceed with a selective reduction (termination of one fetus), the very thought of jeopardizing the pregnancy was extremely frightening. However, we thought about the possibility of one or all of our children being born with autism, cerebral palsy, or other major problems associated with prematurity and knew we should not put them at risk for these complications.

I had to fly to another state to have the termination done with a doctor I did not know, because the procedure is only performed in a few locations nationwide and it wasn't available in our state. The procedure also wasn't covered by my insurance. The center performing the procedure counseled me that I would think about the termination for the rest of my life, and they were right. But, even though I often wonder who our third child could have been, I look at our two healthy children and do not regret the decision.

●

Chapter 12

MENTAL HEALTH RISKS
FOR THE CHILD

In the context of the pathways to parenthood that we're discussing in this book, the possibility of a child having a mental health disorder is a significant concern for many adoptive parents. All parents, however, can benefit from being able to recognize symptoms of mental health difficulties in their children, so you may want to read this chapter even if you aren't considering adoption.

As described in chapter 10, children adopted both domestically and internationally have a higher chance of having been exposed to drugs and alcohol during their birth mother's pregnancy. In addition, many of these children have experienced significant environmental and individual stresses as infants or toddlers. The good news is that after a period of time, most adopted children are well-adjusted, thanks to caring and motivated parents who are attentive to their child's needs. These children seem to catch up to their peers in social, emotional, intellectual, motor, and behavioral competence. The bad news is that some adopted children do not. Despite nurturing parents and unlimited resources, certain mental health disorders, including attachment, sleep, and attention deficit disorders, as well as social maladjustment, are more prevalent among adopted children. Approximately 8 to 10 percent of all patients seen in psychiatric outpatient settings are adopted, making adopted children three to six times more likely than non-adopted children to be referred for psychiatric treatment.

Domestically adopted children have more behavioral and mental health problems than both nonadopted and internationally adopted children. However, internationally adopted children have slightly higher rates of either internalizing their feelings, which tend to be expressed by symptoms of depression or anxiety, or externalizing problems through aggression or hyperactivity. It is still unclear whether internationally adopted boys have more behavioral problems than internationally adopted girls. More girls than boys are adopted, so more research exists for girls.

Despite having fewer behavioral and mental health problems than their domestically adopted peers, internationally adopted children are more likely to receive mental health treatment than both domestically adopted and nonadopted children. This higher treatment rate may be related primarily to the financial well-being of the adoptive parents. The expense of adopting internationally suggests that, on average, these adoptive parents are wealthier and can afford treatment for their children. Adoptive parents in general may be more familiar with social services, having adopted a child. They may also scrutinize their child's behavior more closely and expect more from the child than birth parents would.

In this chapter, we describe the three most prevalent types of mental health disorder—reactive attachment disorder, sleep disorders, and attention deficit/hyperactivity disorder—and available treatments.

REACTIVE ATTACHMENT DISORDER

Most children develop secure attachments to their parents, who respond appropriately, quickly, and consistently to the child's needs while also encouraging independence and exploration. The child, in turn, uses the parents as a secure base in the home environment and effectively copes with stresses. Infants and young children with reactive attachment disorder (RAD) have serious problems with forming emotional attachments and relating socially with their caregivers, family, and peers. Children who lack secure attachments can exhibit a variety of problems, including mistrust and an inability to be emotionally involved with others.

Some of these children are callous and unemotional and as a result they lie and behave badly without later experiencing remorse. They can be aggressive and defiant, and they commonly have low self-esteem or learning disabilities. Developmental delays are also common, and a child lacking a secure attachment may not take part in age-appropriate play activities.

Estimates of the rate of RAD in adopted children range from 10 to 80 percent. Doctors say that parents of children with RAD most often complain that their child is not gaining weight; is detached, unresponsive, and inhibited; is not easily comforted; or does not want to engage in social interactions with others. Conversely, some children with RAD are frequently uninhibited and inappropriately friendly with strangers. Parents may have a hard time reading their child's signals, in part because the child may be giving inconsistent signals about what he or she needs.

Many adoptive parents are unaware of their child's early environmental conditions, but they can be alerted to possible attachment difficulties by several indirect indicators:

- Signs of prior physical abuse, such as old fractures
- Excessive eating or drinking
- Hoarding of food
- Excessive clinginess or withdrawal
- Compressed back of the head, resulting from being left in bed too much

Infants and young children develop attachment problems for a number of reasons, but youngsters at highest risk are those who have been deprived of adequate nutrition and adult attention; have been physically, sexually, or emotionally abused; or have been neglected. Most children develop attachments during their first few years of life, so early changes in caregivers, traumatic losses, and orphanage experiences can disrupt the ability of infants and young children to develop secure attachments. Older adopted children and internationally adopted children are at particular risk. Unfortunately, the time from parental separation to permanent placement with adoptive parents is generally quite long in domestic public agency adoptions, increasing the risk that children will experience negative environmental conditions.

Some of the problems noted in RAD are also seen in other medical conditions, such as disorders of the endocrine and gastrointestinal systems, and in other mental health disorders, including depression, anxiety, and autism. To be sure that the correct diagnosis is made, the child should undergo comprehensive medical and mental health evaluations. If recommended, treatment should be initiated with a competent mental health clinician.

The difficulties a family is having because of symptoms caused by RAD often lead to ineffective parenting practices, and thus the child may have increased behavioral and attitude problems. Because of the ineffective cycle between the behavior of the child and the responses of the parent (and vice versa) prior to beginning treatment, the family must undergo a thorough assessment, not only of the child's aberrant behaviors but also of the child's strengths, the parent's opinions of the child, and the parent's views about discipline and child rearing (among other areas). The targeted treatment that results from this assessment is almost always based on attachment theory and thus involves both the parent (or parents) and the child. Treatment that focuses on the relationship between a pair of individuals is called dyadic therapy.

The goal of dyadic therapy is to build upon the child's and the parent's strengths, to improve interactions between the two, and to develop a healthier parent-child attachment. To achieve these goals, most forms of dyadic therapy involve the therapist observing interactions between the parent and child in different situations (such as at play, in a task the parent is asked to do with the child), teaching parenting skills such as various behavior-management techniques, role-playing between the therapist and the parent, modeling by the therapist with the child, and coaching the parent as he or she interacts with the child. The coaching is often done via a one-way mirror, with the therapist talking to the parent via a bug-in-the-ear; when this technology is not available, the therapist is in the same room as the parent and child. Some examples of dyadic therapy include Parent-Child Interaction Therapy, Developmental Dyadic Therapy, Watch-Wait-and-Wonder, and Floor Time (especially when the child also has developmental delays). The earlier a family enters treatment, the better.

If a child's behaviors involve significant aggression or severe levels of depression, anxiety, or other psychiatric symptoms, individual therapy and/or psychiatric medications may be needed in addition to dyadic therapy. Similarly, because children with RAD often lack the ability to give their parents reciprocal affection, new parents may consider seeking professional emotional support for themselves. Some parents find it helpful to see a therapist, while others attend support groups such as Adoptive Families Together and Parent Network for the Post-Institutionalized Child.

SLEEP DISORDERS

As adults, we have difficulty sleeping in strange places and we are cranky when we don't get enough restful sleep. Children are no different. In most Western cultures, parents separate from their child at bedtime, but many internationally adopted children are not used to sleeping alone, and they also may not be used to sleeping in the dark. Given this, when an adopted child is initially put to bed in his or her nursery and the light is turned off, the child may do anything possible to prevent separation from the parent. If a child is older when adopted, nightmares can be a problem because of early environmental deprivation or an abusive or neglectful background. It may take a while for an adopted child to adapt to new surroundings and sleep situations, but sleep difficulties usually disappear with time. Bedtime routines are essential for all children and should be adhered to without fail with adopted children. If prolonged sleep difficulties occur, professional consultation will be needed.

ATTENTION-DEFICIT/HYPERACTIVITY DISORDER

Most of us have some concept of what attention-deficit/hyperactivity disorder (ADHD) is, and many people probably know a child or adult with ADHD. The most familiar symptoms of ADHD are hyperactivity and impulsivity. Children with these characteristics seem to run before they can walk, cannot sit still, act as if they are driven by a motor, and squirm and wiggle constantly when you can get them to sit in a chair. The side of ADHD we tend to be less familiar with is the inattention. Children with ADHD who are inattentive cannot stay focused on one activity, do not seem to listen, are easily bored, are forgetful, or daydream. They sometimes fall through the cracks because they don't act up like their hyperactive peers.

Although ADHD is not usually diagnosed until age five or six years, the American Academy of Child and Adolescent Psychiatry indicates that symptoms of ADHD can be identified as early as infancy. Symptoms include sleeping very little or for short periods of time, being demanding, poor sucking, crying during feedings, needing to be fed often for brief periods, irritability, fidgeting, crying, or resistance to being held. Infants may soothe themselves with excessive thumb sucking, head rolling, head banging, or rocking.

Approximately 3 to 7 percent of school-age children are estimated to have ADHD. The rate of ADHD in adopted children is higher, with estimates ranging from 20 to 40 percent. ADHD is considered to be largely a hereditary disorder of the nervous system. Genetic factors are thought to account for 70 to 95 percent of the characteristics displayed by a child with ADHD, but other factors are also involved, including family environment, parenting, peer relationships, and diet. The increased rate of ADHD in adopted children may be due to preadoption abuse or neglect, prenatal drug or alcohol exposure, high lead levels (both prenatal exposure and current high blood levels), malnutrition, or infection of the central nervous system.

For ADHD to be diagnosed, a child must be hyperactive or inattentive or both. These symptoms must disrupt the child's life to the point of causing problems with social relations, education, family function, self-sufficiency, or adherence to rules and norms.

Table 12.1. Behaviors Seen in People with Attention-Deficit/Hyperactivity Disorder (ADHD)

Behavior	Percentage of people with ADHD exhibiting the behavior
Drops out of school	32–40
Has few or no friends	50–70
Underperforms at work	70–80
Engages in antisocial activities	40–50
Becomes pregnant as a teen	40
Contracts sexually transmitted diseases	16
Experiences depression as an adult	20–30
Has a personality disorder as an adult	18–25

Source: International Consensus Statement on ADHD, January 2002. *Clin Child Fam Psychol Rev* 2002;5:89–111.

Research indicates that individuals with ADHD are at increased risk for the behavioral difficulties listed in table 12.1.

Fewer than half of individuals with ADHD receive treatment. Yet ADHD is a highly treatable disorder. Strict behavior-management programs are necessary in the home and at school. Cognitive Behavior Therapy, social skills training, parent training, family therapy, and medications may also be needed in some cases. Parents, the child with ADHD, and the child's peers and teachers are all equally important in the comprehensive treatment of this disorder. Parents should become educated about ADHD and serve as advocates for their children, to ensure that they are getting all the services that will help them manage their ADHD. Other mental health disorders can coexist with ADHD.

Other conditions can be mistaken for ADHD. For example, impaired vision or hearing, seizures, acute or chronic medical illnesses, poor nutrition, and insufficient sleep share some of the signs and symptoms of ADHD. A thorough pediatric evaluation will ensure a correct diagnosis.

POSITIVE ASPECTS TO CONSIDER

- If you choose a fertility assisted option, you need not worry about a higher than average risk of mental health disorders in your child.
- If you choose to adopt, you have the opportunity to make a big difference in a child's life by offering the child love, a nurturing environment, medical and mental health care, and educational opportunities.
- Adopted children have often undergone great stresses during their short lives, and many of them develop a special resilience that will most likely benefit them in dealing with future adverse events.

FURTHER READING

American Academy of Child and Adolescent Psychiatry (an organization that addresses reactive attachment disorder and other mental health issues). www.aacap.org.

J. D. Osofsky, ed. *Young Children and Trauma: Intervention and Treatment.* Guilford Press, 2004.

D. B. Pruitt and American Academy of Child and Adolescent Psychiatry, eds. *Your Child: What Every Parent Needs to Know about Childhood Development from Birth to Preadolescence.* HarperCollins, 1998 (hardback), 2000 (paperback).

C. H. Zeanah Jr., ed. *Handbook of Infant Mental Health.* 2nd ed. Guilford Press, 2000.

I AM A LESBIAN in my late forties. I never even considered parenthood until age forty. When I came out, in the mid-1970s, gay parenthood was not the norm; in fact, it seemed an oddity to me. In the last decade, however, it's become much more common for gay people to raise children. This openness made it easier for me when I decided I would like to be a mother.

I decided to adopt an eighteen-month-old girl from China, which felt like a totally natural choice. I had never wanted to go through child-birth, and I felt that I was making a meaningful contribution to society by adopting a Chinese girl who otherwise would have had a childhood of institutional life with little education or future prospects.

For me, the hardest part of the adoption was not knowing if my child would be healthy, not only physically, but emotionally and mentally as well. My daughter did have giardia, an intestinal parasite infection that was easily treated. Of more concern, however, was the fact that she seemed overly active. As time went on, it became clear that she had ADHD. After about five years on medication, she got to the point where it was impossible to get her to take her medication. This struggle turned out to be worse than the condition itself. My daughter has been off med-ication for a while now and has done relatively well.

At nine years old, my daughter is smart (in the gifted program at school), well-adjusted, sweet, and funny—everything I would ever want her to be.

I feared the day that she realized being adopted also meant that her birth mother had given her away. But since I have been open and hon-est from the beginning, it hasn't been as devastating as it could have been. I have always focused on the loving, difficult choice her birth mother made in the face of adversity.

The international adoption process took me about a year and a half to complete. Although this seems like a long time, the end result has been worth every minute of the wait. I have gone from being a person who never considered parenthood to one who is a fervent supporter of adoption.

In retrospect, the only thing I would have done differently is not to have taken so long to decide to become a parent. My daughter is the best thing that has ever happened to me.

Chapter 13

EMOTIONAL COSTS

What You Might Experience

Without doubt, parenting can be both emotionally rewarding and emotionally draining, and for some of us, the roller coaster ride starts long before we bring a baby or child home. Making the decision to start a family is exciting. If you have difficulty conceiving, though, the excitement can quickly turn to frustration, sadness, and anxiety. Events such as miscarriage, stillbirth, and birth defects bring out a host of other emotions, including grief, guilt, and anger. Sometimes things go wrong in surrogacy arrangements or adoptions, and the prospective parents are left without the baby or child they thought they would bring home.

When, finally, a baby or child is on the way, whether through fertility assisted pregnancy, surrogacy, or adoption, still more emotions and concerns come flooding in. A worry common to many prospective parents is whether their baby or child will love them and, conversely, whether they will love their baby or child. These fears may be more intense the more genetically removed a parent is from the child and, in the case of adoptions, the older the child.

Nothing can really prepare you for the emotional journey you will face as you follow your chosen pathway to parenthood. Everyone's experience will be a little different, and everyone will react to and cope with situations in different ways. Nevertheless, it may help to be aware of some of the situations that can occur so that, at the least, you know you aren't alone in experiencing the lows (and, of course, the highs) of trying to achieve parenthood.

In this chapter, we discuss emotional factors that you may want to consider for both the short term, while you're trying to become a parent, and the long term, when you are raising your child or children.

FERTILITY ASSISTANCE

Beginning the fertility workup after an unsuccessful period of trying to conceive can be a huge relief. At long last some progress is being made, even if it is only to find out why you have been unsuccessful. As an individual or couple goes through the various tests in the fertility workup, the doctor may find an explanation for their infertility. Having a specific reason why you aren't able to conceive can be wonderful news, especially if the problem is correctable. On the other hand, some diagnoses may be difficult to deal with, such as finding a genetic defect or discovering that the male partner does not have any sperm. Yet simply having a diagnosis helps many people move on, either to address the problem or to follow a new pathway. Some people complete the fertility workup and are left without an answer; a diagnosis of unexplained infertility can be both bewildering and frustrating. Still, it may help these people to know that they have nothing specifically wrong and that they have a reasonable chance of conceiving with just a small amount of assistance.

A large part of fertility assistance, both early assistance procedures and assisted reproductive technologies (ART), involves hormonal manipulation. Hormones can have side effects of headache, bloating, weight gain, and mood swings. For many women, the hormone variations over the natural monthly cycle cause these side effects. With hormonal manipulation, however, the levels of some hormones can go much higher than they normally do, so even women who aren't usually affected by their monthly hormone changes can find themselves dealing with side effects when they undergo hormone treatment. Some women are particularly prone

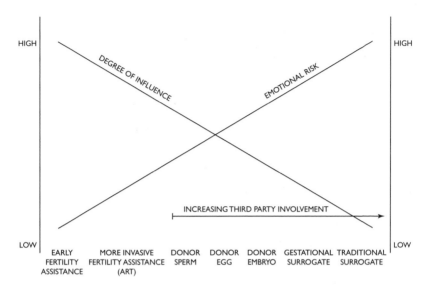

Figure 13.1. Degree of control and emotional risk with different pathways to parenthood.

to the side effects and may suffer depression (or euphoria) purely due to the hormonal influences. Fortunately, the side effects go away when the hormone treatment stops.

Most fertility assistance options require that specific tests, procedures, and interventions be done at specific times. Many people find it stressful to make sure that they are in the right place and doing the right thing at the right time. Obviously, timing is critical for conception through fertility assistance. Some men find it exceedingly difficult, if not impossible, to perform on demand in an unfamiliar environment when they must produce their sperm sample. The expectations are high when a man's partner has been jabbing herself with needles for over a week in preparation for an intrauterine insemination (IUI) or an in vitro fertilization (IVF) procedure. There are ways around all difficulties, though, including a man's inability to perform at the right time. Although fresh sperm are ideal, it is possible to provide sperm samples ahead of time for freezing, just in case they're needed.

Going through fertility assistance can also have an impact on a couple's sex life. Depending on the procedure, a couple will be instructed on when during the process to have and not to have intercourse. The scheduling obviously removes any spontaneity and can become a strain on a couple's relationship.

For many people, the emotional cost of using fertility procedures rises with the procedures' increasing complexity, invasiveness, and use of third party assistance. As figure 13.1 shows, the emotional toll tends to go up as the degree of control goes down. For other people, the excitement and optimism remain and even increase with each new attempt or procedure. A cyclic emotional response, illustrated in figure 13.2, is fairly typical. Hopes build

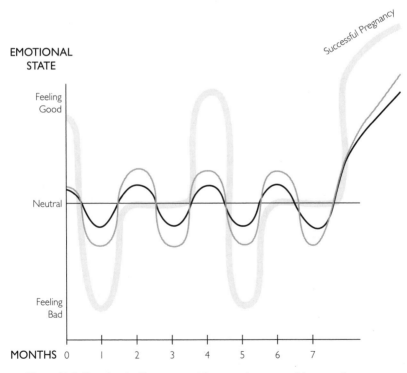

Figure 13.2. Emotional roller coaster with repeated unsuccessful conception attempts. Thin black line: no or minimal fertility assistance; thin gray line: more aggressive fertility assistance such as hormone stimulation; thick gray line: assisted reproductive technology assistance or in vitro fertilization attempts.

up as each attempt progresses, and if it isn't successful, the hopes crash quickly and the couple is distraught. The degree by which hopes rise and fall gets larger as increasingly invasive assistance is used. For women, some of the emotional crash can be attributed to the sudden decline in hormone levels as the body rids itself of the uterine lining that was supposed to support the pregnancy.

All fertility centers have psychologists or counselors on staff or can refer you to such a professional. These counselors can help prepare you for the emotions you may experience during fertility assistance procedures, and they can also help you work through your feelings and reconsider your options if one or several attempts at pregnancy don't work.

UNPLANNED EVENTS

If a woman or a couple successfully achieves pregnancy with fertility assistance, they may ride an emotional high for the entire pregnancy. The pregnancy-related discomforts can be comforting to a woman by reminding her of her success. Of course, many people have already experienced miscarriage and other setbacks on their journey to parenthood, and they may remain both cautious and anxious throughout the pregnancy. At first the anxiety centers on carrying the pregnancy through the first trimester, when miscarriage rates are highest, and then on continuing the pregnancy to a point where the fetus could survive, albeit with medical interventions (at about 21 weeks), and finally on completing the pregnancy without complications.

For some people who become pregnant and experience the awe and excitement of seeing a positive pregnancy test, the dream, sadly, does not come true. Miscarriage claims some of these pregnancies and leaves the parents grief stricken, and often angry or even feeling guilty that they have somehow caused the miscarriage. Miscarriages, especially first-trimester miscarriages, usually happen because of a chromosomal abnormality or other problem with the fetus. A woman who miscarries is not at fault for causing the miscarriage and must try to accept that it's a natural event.

She and her partner will grieve and should allow themselves to do so, because no matter how far along the pregnancy was, they have lost a baby. The grief will lessen with time, and for some people with professional counseling. Then they must move on and try to conceive again, try a different pathway to parenthood, or decide not to pursue parenthood.

Sometimes, the woman or couple decides to undergo chorionic villus sampling (CVS) or amniocentesis (both discussed in chapter 10), and then they receive the heartbreaking news that the fetus has a debilitating defect or condition. The condition may be so severe that the fetus is unlikely to survive the pregnancy or, if it does, the baby will not survive its first few hours, days, or months of life. In these situations, the parents must decide whether to undergo an elective abortion or to allow nature to take its course. People who decide to abort the pregnancy will undoubtedly feel a tremendous sense of loss, and they may be plagued with thoughts about whether they made the right decision. As with miscarriages, they must allow themselves the time to grieve the loss and then look forward to their next attempt at achieving parenthood.

A stillbirth occurs when a fetus lives beyond 20 weeks gestation and then dies. Though rare, stillbirths do happen, and frequently the cause is unknown. Being the parent of a stillborn baby is utterly devastating. There are organizations and support groups that parents in this situation can join to help them deal with their emotions.

When a woman or couple finally achieves pregnancy with fertility assistance, they begin to imagine what their baby will look like. They are unlikely to imagine their baby with a birth defect, so if the baby is born with one, it will be a shock. Birth defects range from potentially severe disabilities, such as cystic fibrosis or muscular dystrophy, to relatively minor problems, such as a club foot or cleft lip. Not all birth defects are visible ones—for example, heart defects—and some may develop later in life, such as porphyria (a blood disorder). Many of the more minor defects can be fairly easily corrected or alleviated and the child will live a completely normal life. Even babies with more severe birth defects, such as Down syndrome, can lead full and productive lives. When parents first learn that their baby has a birth defect, they may feel sad or angry and they may worry that they won't be able to fully love the child. Others may feel protective and defensive. All of these reactions are normal because it's an adjustment for parents to come to terms with the knowledge that they don't have the "perfect" baby they had envisioned before birth. Again, there are numerous organizations that provide information, advice, and support to families dealing with birth defects.

Postpartum depression can occur soon after or several months after a woman gives birth. In addition to the feelings of sadness, hopelessness, and guilt that the mother may experience, she may be troubled by why she is suffering postpartum depression when she so desperately wanted a child. Any mother with postpartum depression needs to receive professional help to get better.

MULTIPLE GESTATIONS

The joy at becoming pregnant after fertility assistance or ART can be dampened by worry if the pregnancy has multiple fetuses. Most people would probably be delighted to learn that they were pregnant with twins; twin pregnancies generally have a good outcome even though risks are higher than with a singleton pregnancy (as discussed in chapter 11). However, triplets and higher-order pregnancies have a greater risk of complications and therefore cause additional anxiety for the parents. As well as anxiety about the pregnancy itself and the health of the babies at birth, many people will be anxious about parenting several children of the same age and about coping financially.

Parents of multiples face numerous challenges that can take an emotional toll on themselves, their relationship with each other, and their family. The American Society for Reproductive Medicine lists the following psychological and social challenges:

- Multiples may be hard to tell apart, even if they are not identical.

- Parents may bond to multiples differently than they would to single-born children.
- Managing the physical care of multiples, particularly in early infancy and childhood, is more demanding than managing singletons.
- Parents of multiples may feel socially isolated, given the lack of personal time, the demands of parenthood, and the financial costs.
- Multiples often attract unwanted attention.
- Older siblings may have problems adjusting to multiples.
- The financial impact may be substantial (see chapter 16).
- Compared with a singleton birth, the health care cost for delivery and newborn care is fourfold higher for twins and twelve-fold higher for triplets.

When a multiple pregnancy is confirmed, the parents have the option of undergoing a selective reduction. They will, of course, pay an emotional cost in contemplating whether or not to go through with the procedure, undergoing the procedure itself, and thinking about the result after the procedure. If the whole pregnancy miscarries after the procedure, the parents may blame themselves, each other, or the physician. They will most likely feel a broad sweep of emotions as they deal with shifting from the thought of having several babies at once to not being pregnant at all. Counseling is available at centers offering selective reduction services to help people deal with these emotions and thoughts. In considering whether to undergo the procedure, people should think about the advantage to the surviving fetuses. The benefit is particularly pronounced for pregnancies with quadruplets or more, primarily because of the prolonged gestational length for the surviving fetuses.

USING A DONOR

Many people who decide to pursue donor sperm, eggs, or embryos feel some relief in knowing that their chances for successful conception are probably higher than with their own gametes. Some women who have been through unsuccessful IVF treatments are also pleasantly surprised that donor egg assistance can be easier, because they don't have to undergo the hormone stimulation themselves. Of course, there are still many emotions involved in deciding to use a donor and in having a baby with donor assistance. For example, when one partner in a couple is genetically related to the child and the other isn't, the partner who is not related may feel inadequate or unequal. Also, a single woman who uses an anonymous sperm donor won't have a father's name to write on the child's birth certificate, which may make her feel a stigma of illegitimacy.

Deciding which donor to use can be an emotionally draining process because the decision will make such a difference to the genetic makeup of the child. After finally deciding on a donor and attempting pregnancy, it may be necessary to change to another donor if further sperm samples or eggs are unavailable or if several attempts have been unsuccessful.

Individuals and couples opting for egg or sperm donation may agonize over whether to pursue a known versus an anonymous donor. Using a known donor usually means having more information about the donor's family history, but using an anonymous donor gives some people stronger feelings of possession, as discussed by Susan Cooper and Ellen Glazer in their book *Beyond Infertility*. If there is an established relationship between a known donor and a child's family, the child may be confused about who his or her real parents are.

People who successfully conceive and have a baby with donor gametes must decide how much of the child's origins to disclose and to whom. People who decide to keep their child's origins secret and who aren't genetically related to the child need to be prepared to handle comments such as, "Your baby looks just like you." Family members or friends may discuss the child's resemblance to other family members. On the other hand, people who are open about using donor sperm or eggs may find that they are asked personal questions that invade their privacy.

USING A SURROGATE

Many people struggle with the idea of having to ask someone else to do something as personal as carry and give birth to their child, and some women are troubled by not being able to experience pregnancy. But, as with deciding to use a donor, other people may feel relieved that they are moving on to a pathway that has a good chance of success. Some women may also be relieved to avoid the unpleasant aspects of pregnancy.

Once they've decided to pursue a surrogacy arrangement, the individual or couple must decide what type it will be, traditional or gestational surrogacy (see chapter 6 for a discussion of these types). Their decision may come down to how concerned they are about the surrogate deciding to retain custody of the child after its birth. Even though, in traditional surrogacy, the intended father, whose sperm was used for the pregnancy, is also the legal father, the surrogate has the right to decide to keep the child. During the pregnancy and at the baby's birth, the traditional surrogate is the legal mother because her eggs were used for the pregnancy. Therefore, the surrogate must give up her right to legal custody and the intended mother must adopt the child. Unfortunately, surrogates can change their mind and may choose not to honor any agreements made prior to the pregnancy.

The intended parents can't be assured that transition of the baby to them will go smoothly until the final court appearance has been completed after the child's birth. There are steps that can be taken when finding and working with a traditional surrogate to minimize the chances of the surrogate deciding to keep the baby, but it can nevertheless be a stressful wait for the final documents to be signed. Two steps that help in setting up a successful surrogacy arrangement are, first, to use a large and respected agency with strong legal representation that does thorough and strict screening of surrogates and, second, to use a surrogate living in a state that recognizes and permits surrogacy. People who find a surrogate online or elsewhere and don't have the opportunity to thor-

oughly screen and get to know her may not discover any potential mental health issues that could increase the risk of the arrangement falling through.

Using a gestational surrogate avoids the risk of the surrogate
deciding to keep the baby. Because a gestational surrogate does
not use her own eggs for the pregnancy, the intended parents are
usually considered the legal parents of the child from the moment
of conception.

Once the decision has been made to use a traditional or gestational surrogate, the intended parents need to find a surrogate they
are comfortable with and feel they can trust. Many people worry
that a surrogate may engage in behaviors that could harm the baby,
and they feel frustrated or even frightened at not having control
of the fetal environment. They may also be concerned about building a good relationship with the surrogate; they want to be close
to her, but not too close, because the relationship could affect future contact.

People who enter surrogacy arrangements of either type will
find themselves dealing with a range of emotions and issues. For
example, they will need to be prepared for rumors, sometimes even
from within their own families, that they are buying a baby. After the baby's birth, people who don't know about the surrogacy
may comment on how good the new mother looks so soon after
the birth. Such comments, innocent though they may be, can be
hard to hear and respond to.

ADOPTION

Deciding to adopt a child is a wonderful feeling. You know that
you'll have the opportunity to raise a child and make a difference
in the child's life. Going through the adoption process can be
lengthy, however, and many people find that they experience both
highs and lows before they finally bring a child home.

One of the first things to happen after submitting the initial
application is the home study. A home study is required for all
types of adoption and can be stressful, because it is so detailed and

the questions can be very personal. The applicants may have several visits with the social worker before the recommendation is made that they are suitable (or unsuitable, of course) to be adoptive parents. People often find that a layer of anxiety is lifted from them when they pass the hurdle of the home study.

In both domestic and international agency adoptions, long periods can go by with little or no information about the progress of the application and how soon a child may be available. This waiting game can fray nerves and increase anxieties. For some people, the wait is relatively short, but for others it can be several months or even longer. When a child is identified, the prospective parents will probably be filled with both joy and anticipation, although they're likely to remain a little cautious as well until they've had a chance to review the child's medical report and decide if this child is the one they will welcome into their family. Preparing to meet and then meeting the child can be nerve-wracking for some people. They will be filled with many emotions, including excitement, joy, nervousness, and maybe even a little bit of fear. If all goes well, though, the adoptive parents bring their child home and parents and child begin to get to know each other. The adoptive parents may feel a great sense of relief that they've successfully navigated the adoption process and can now focus on building family bonds.

Domestic Adoptions

Finding a Birth Mother

People who want to adopt a baby at or soon after birth have a few options. They can go to an agency that matches infants with adoptive parents or that allows the adoptive parents to find a birth mother themselves. They can also decide to pursue an independent adoption. These options are discussed in chapter 7. If the prospective parents are responsible for finding the birth mother, they must effectively sell themselves. It can be very stressful for people to put together a portfolio that they think will present themselves in the best possible light. They may be concerned about how they look, how much money they make, and what type of life they can offer a child.

When an agency is involved, birth mothers contact the agency directly. In an independent adoption, the prospective parents must find the birth mother themselves, which they may do by advertising (if it's legal to do so in their state). People who advertise need to provide their contact information and must be prepared to receive phone calls from birth mothers. One recommended tactic is to have a separate phone line on which to receive these calls. Unfortunately, prank calls may be received as well. Over the period of a year, as many as 50 birth mothers may phone to interview the prospective parents. Most birth mothers interview several families, though, and only 1 in 10 initial calls results in an adoption. The prospective parents will invest emotional energy into each of the calls they receive, yet the investment may not pay off. Nevertheless, they must try to remain positive and keep up their hopes, because eventually one of the calls will pay off, and they never know which call it will be.

Adoption Disruption

The term "adoption disruption" refers to an adoption process that stops after a child is placed into an adoptive home and before the adoption is finalized legally. In any type of domestic adoption in which the birth mother, birth parents, or legal guardians have a choice, they may change their minds at any time before signing the papers to relinquish the child. Adoptive parents may also change their minds; the child then returns to the birth parents, goes to foster care, or is placed with new adoptive parents. Adoption disruption can occur with both infants and older children being adopted through either private or public agencies.

Although fewer than 1 percent of infant adoptions disrupt, with children older than age three and with special needs children, 10 to 15 percent of adoptions disrupt. When infant adoptions disrupt, the birth mother most often changes her mind within the 48 hours prior to or after the birth. In contrast, adoption disruptions with older children generally occur because the adoptive par-

ANXIETY

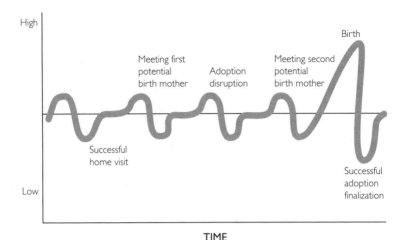

Figure 13.3. Emotional roller coaster in open adoptions.

ents no longer feel they can parent the child. Factors that are associated with adoption disruption include the number of foster care placements the child has experienced, the behavioral and emotional needs of the child, and agency staff turnover.

Losing an adoption because the birth mother or birth parents change their mind has been likened to losing a pregnancy. The adoptive parents prepare physically, emotionally, and mentally for the arrival of their child, so they feel an extreme sense of loss if the child they have been thinking about for weeks or months does not arrive. Figure 13.3 illustrates anxiety levels for parents faced with adoption disruption in an open adoption. Only one type of domestic adoption—a closed adoption—protects the prospective parents from the emotional risk of an adoption disruption caused by the birth mother or birth parents. In a closed adoption, the prospective parents are not contacted until the birth mother or birth parents have signed the final papers, as shown in figure 13.4.

Having an adoption disrupt due to the unexpected challenges of parenting an older child or one with special needs can also be highly stressful. Adoptive parents can experience feelings of in-

ANXIETY

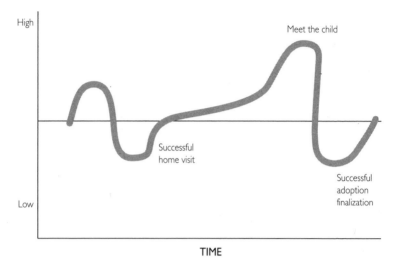

Figure 13.4. Emotional roller coaster in closed adoptions.

adequacy, failure, and guilt. These feelings can be so overwhelming that the adoptive parents may opt not to pursue a subsequent adoption.

Adoption Dissolution

The term "adoption dissolution" refers to an adoption that ends after it has been legally finalized. In most states, the legal documents signed by a birth mother or birth parents are irrevocable. However, the birth parents can go through a court process to try to obtain their biological child. Fewer than 2 percent of birth parents change their mind after signing the legal papers, and fewer than 0.1 percent of adoptions are contested in court.

Birth Fathers Asserting Parental Rights

In about 1 of every 100 domestic adoptions, the father will try to assert his parental rights. Sometimes the birth father's feelings about the adoption are unknown until the baby is placed with adoptive parents. Birth fathers can try to block or at least delay any attempt by the birth mother to place a child for adoption, but few are successful. Several states have putative father registries where unmarried men who believe they have fathered a child can register their paternity. In some states, if a birth father has not registered, the birth mother can place her child for adoption without taking any additional action. In other states, an effort must be made to try to find the birth father and let him know of the child's birth. State laws vary as to what happens if a birth mother does not know who the birth father is, or if she refuses to name him. She may have to tell the judge why she can't or won't name the birth father, or it may be left up to the father to register in the putative father registry or to come forward if he wants to assert his parental rights.

Short Notice about an Available Infant or Child

In independent adoptions and open adoptions through a private agency, the prospective parents generally know when they can expect their child to arrive. They can prepare themselves both at home and at work for the day when they bring the child home. On the other hand, with public agency and closed adoptions, the prospective parents may get very little notice that a child is available and ready to come to their home. It is not unusual for people to be called by the agency with the news that an infant or child will be available the next day. The adoptive parents are given medical information on the child, but they may have very little time—as little as a few hours or a day—to review it and make their decision to accept or decline the child. Clearly, this situation is both joyful and stressful.

Deciding Whether to Adopt a Special Needs Child

Some people decide that they are willing to adopt a child with special needs and they are expecting such a child. Many children adopted from a public agency have special needs. People who are unsure whether they would be willing to adopt a child with special needs may find it least distressing to work with a closed adoption. In a closed adoption, the prospective parents don't meet the birth mother or birth parents and therefore don't form any sort of relationship with them. If an infant or child with special needs or medical conditions becomes available, the prospective parents can make their decision privately. The prospective parents may feel less anxiety about declining an adoption because they won't have had contact with the birth mother or been involved during the pregnancy. The decision will undoubtedly be a difficult one for many people who have been waiting to adopt a child, and they may feel frustrated to find themselves in the position of having to decide whether they can commit to a child with special needs. On the other hand, some prospective parents feel that they have the emotional and financial capacity to welcome a special needs child into their family and offer the child the best possible chance of living with or overcoming the condition.

In an open adoption, the prospective parents have formed some kind of relationship with the birth mother. They may have met the birth mother only briefly, or they may have gotten to know her well. In the case of an independent adoption, they will have supported the birth mother throughout her pregnancy. If she then gives birth to a child with birth defects or other medical problems, the prospective parents will have to decide in a limited time, usually a few days, whether they wish to finalize the adoption. The decision can be a traumatic one to have to make. Some agencies may have counselors available to discuss the situation with the parents. There is no right or wrong decision, because all adoptive parents are different and have different abilities to care for a special needs child.

International Adoptions

There is little possibility of an international adoption being disrupted by the birth parents, because children available for adoption are generally considered to be orphans in their birth country. Their birth parents have already made the decision to relinquish their parental rights, and the risk of a birth mother or birth father later trying to claim the child is virtually zero. A situation sometimes occurs, however, where an individual or couple is interested in adopting a certain child but the orphanage has promised this child to several agencies. The orphanage's goal is to place children as quickly as possible.

Short notice is another problem that will not arise with an international adoption done through a reputable agency. Usually, an available child is proposed to the prospective parents and they then decide if they will go ahead with adopting the child. The length of time available to accept or decline a proposed child depends on both the agency and the country involved. Making the decision may be difficult for some people, depending on how much information they receive.

Sometimes, though rarely, political relationships and threats of terrorist activities can jeopardize international adoptions during the proceedings. As of December 2007, the U.S. Department of State had a travel warning for Guatemala because of violent criminal activity. Adoptions can also be suspended because of suspected child trafficking. For example, as of December 2007, all international adoptions from Lesotho, including adoptions in progress by American citizens, were suspended for this reason. The date when these adoptions can resume is unknown. At any time a country may decide to suspend all adoptions, usually temporarily. Adoptions that are in progress, particularly those in the early stages, are stopped until the country reopens its adoptions. For example, in April 2007 Ukraine suspended new applications for three weeks because of staffing shortages. Another example is that the Memorandum of Agreement with Vietnam for adoptions expired in September 2008. In addition, several serious adoption irregularities have recently been noted for this country.

With international adoptions, there is also a risk that a child has a medical condition or other problem that the adoptive parents were not told about. Unfortunately, medical records are generally limited and are in a foreign language. Although some countries provide pictures or videos of children awaiting adoption, many adoptive parents see their child for the first time when they meet in the child's birth country. Generally, legal proceedings can be stopped and the child declined. This situation would be emotionally difficult to deal with, especially with the excitement of having traveled to bring a child home.

COMMON EMOTIONAL ISSUES

Bonding with Your Child

Although some people may believe that individuals not related by blood will never feel totally connected, the reality is that parents generally bond with their child over time through caring for and loving the child. Bonding or attachment is not usually an issue for children conceived through donor sperm, eggs, or embryos. However, it may be a concern for parents who adopt, particularly for those adopting children past the baby stage who have already developed a personality and habits, and who may understand or speak a different language. In these cases, bonding is a process that can take up to five years. It is important for at least one parent to spend up to six months at home after the adoption to initiate the bonding process before returning to work.

Disclosing Your Child's Origins

People who choose to have a child with donor sperm, eggs, or embryos or choose to adopt need to decide how much information they want to share with the child about his or her origins. The American Society for Reproductive Medicine provides a list of points for and against disclosure to a child.

Considerations for disclosure are:

- Humans have a fundamental interest in and perhaps even a legal right to know about their biological origins.
- Disclosure is an important part of open and honest communication with children.
- Planned disclosure will protect the child from accidentally finding out about his or her origins.

- There can be a medical advantage to knowing about genetic risks for specific health problems.
- Disclosure can protect against later inadvertent romantic relationships between blood-related relatives.

Considerations against disclosure are:

- The child may be subject to social and psychological turmoil.
- A child conceived with donor sperm or a donor egg differs from an adopted child in that one parent is genetically related to the child.

When parents do tell their children about how they were conceived or that they were adopted, a child will ask questions—perhaps not right away, but eventually. The parents may feel guilty when their child pressures them for more details about his or her biological parents and they don't have the answers. It can be hard to see a child experience frustration, sadness, and anger over a lack of information about his or her origins. Adopted children and children conceived with assistance from a third party may also try to use this information to hurt their parents when they are angry. For example, some children will tell their parents that they aren't their real parents.

Children conceived with donor sperm or eggs can feel as if they are adopted and often go through the same emotions as adopted children. In *Raising Adopted Children*, Louis Melina discusses how adopted children will struggle to make sense of what it means to be adopted. Adopted children deal with a variety of emotions, including grief, loss, and rejection, as well as issues of identity, intimacy, and lack of control. Adolescents need to form an identity twice, once in relation to their adoptive family and again in relation to their biological family. They may wonder why their biological parents did not raise them; they may worry that something was wrong with them. They may even have concerns about their adoptive parents giving them up. That adopted children experience these emotions and face these issues does not mean they have pathological disorders, but they will probably want to talk about their feelings at some point and the parents need to be ready for the discussion.

Researchers who have studied adopted children have found that secrecy about a child's origins often damages the child. The child feels betrayed when the truth eventually comes out, and sometimes a child believes there is something wrong about having been adopted. Policies about the anonymity of sperm and egg donors may follow the trend of adoption regulations, which have now shifted toward greater openness whereby birth parents agree to being contacted when a child grows up.

POSITIVE ASPECTS TO CONSIDER

- Raising a child is a rewarding experience. Most people with children say the best thing they ever did was to have a family.
- If you choose fertility assistance and become pregnant, you may be overjoyed to experience pregnancy.
- If you choose surrogacy or adoption, you may be relieved not to experience pregnancy.
- If you are over thirty-five years old and elect to use donor eggs or embryos, you will lessen your concerns about chromosomal abnormalities and you won't need an amniocentesis.
- If you choose adoption and have concerns about a child's special needs, you can change your mind prior to finalizing the adoption.
- Domestic public agency and international adoptions have a low risk of adoption disruption, and you also avoid stresses such as finding a birth mother and maintaining a good relationship with her.
- If you adopt, you have the opportunity to make a real difference in a child's life.

FURTHER READING

H. Aizley. *Buying Dad: One Woman's Search for the Perfect Sperm Donor.* Alyson Publications, 2003.

S. Cooper and E. Glazer. *Beyond Infertility: The New Paths to Parenthood.* Lexington Books, 1994.

D. Ehrensaft. *Mommies, Daddies, Donors, Surrogates: Answering Tough Questions and Building Strong Families.* Guilford Press, 2005.

L. R. Melina. *Raising Adopted Children.* Rev. ed. HarperCollins, 1998.

● ──

MY HUSBAND AND I GOT MARRIED very young. We wanted a big family and we liked the idea of having our kids while we were young, so we immediately stopped using birth control. I didn't get pregnant right away, but it was okay because my husband was still studying and it would have been hard financially if I was home caring for a baby instead of working. Three years later my husband had graduated and started working and we still weren't pregnant. We went to a doctor and all the tests he did came back with normal results. He suggested that we try some fertility medications. We felt conflicted; on the one hand we wanted to have children while we were young, and on the other hand we really didn't want to have outside help. We didn't want to mess with nature, so we decided that we'd keep trying on our own, and at the same time we'd start looking into adoption. This was a hard time for our relationship, but somehow we got through it and accepted the fact that we would have to build our family with adoption.

We went for an international adoption from China, because my mother is Chinese. A little over a year after starting the process, we adopted a fourteen-month-old baby girl. It was so wonderful to finally be parents! Six months after our daughter came home, we started the adoption process again. The second adoption was completed a little faster and we adopted a nine-month-old girl. Our two-and-a-half-year-old was delighted with her younger sister.

To our shock and amazement, the month after we brought our second daughter home, I became pregnant. I could hardly believe it! In fact, it felt a bit strange because I had long since given up the thought of having biological children. I even felt somehow betrayed by my body, but once I got over these emotions I became excited about adding a third child to our family. We now have three daughters. We've decided not to adopt any more children, but we still don't use birth control, so if I happen to get pregnant again we'd feel blessed to welcome a fourth child into our family.

Chapter 14

TIME COSTS

How Long before You Become a Parent?

We know that many readers of this book will want to become a parent immediately, and some, especially women over thirty-five years of age, will feel an intense sense of urgency. No matter which pathway you choose to become a parent, you will need patience. None of the options will make you a parent overnight. For most options, it typically takes at least a year, possibly longer, to bring a baby or child home. During this time, taking vacations or leaving town may be difficult, particularly if you are pursuing fertility assistance.

In this chapter, we outline how long it can take to become a parent with fertility assistance, surrogacy, and adoption. The range is large, of course. Some people are fortunate enough to become pregnant on their first attempt at a fertility center or to find a birth mother within days of starting their search. Other people endure attempt after attempt at pregnancy or make progress initially and then suffer a setback. There are no guarantees, but with perseverance and a positive attitude, virtually everyone who wants to be a parent does eventually fulfill this dream.

HOW LONG DOES IT TAKE TO GET PREGNANT WITH FERTILITY ASSISTANCE?

Every fertility center has a different waiting time for the initial consultation with a fertility specialist, but in general the wait can be a few weeks to a few months. The fertility workup can also take as long as several months, depending on the woman's or couple's fertility history and the type of tests the specialist orders. Once the evaluation has been completed, the time it takes to conceive will depend in part on the treatment chosen and in part on the woman's age. As discussed earlier in the book, maternal age is one of the key factors in a woman's chances of conceiving and carrying a pregnancy to term. Older women, on average, need to undergo more cycles to achieve a pregnancy. Younger women are more fertile and have a higher chance of conception with each cycle they attempt. They also have more child-bearing time still available to them. Therefore, fertility specialists usually recommend that women in their twenties try less aggressive treatments for a longer time and that women in their late thirties or early forties move more quickly to the more aggressive treatments. For example, a twenty-five-year-old woman may be counseled to continue trying hormone stimulation with intrauterine insemination (IUI) for a year, whereas a thirty-eight-year-old woman may be advised to move on to in vitro fertilization (IVF) treatment after a limited number of unsuccessful early assistance attempts.

Using Your Own Eggs and Sperm

Women who begin fertility treatment with early assistance methods such as Clomid or hormone stimulation should discuss the recommended number of cycles with their doctor. Clomid can continue to be taken for consecutive cycles if the woman doesn't conceive. Generally, though, doctors will move on to other treatments if conception is not successful after three to six cycles. With the injectable hormones used in hormone stimulation treatments, women may be advised to rest for one or two months between treatment cycles to give the body time to recuperate from the hormone shifts. Therefore, in a 12-month period, there may be only five or six attempted cycles. Sometimes, women who have experienced years of infertility try one or several hormone stimulation cycles, don't conceive, take a month off before the next treatment cycle, and then find to their astonishment that they've conceived naturally during the month off.

Many women and couples who have moved on to assisted reproductive technology (ART) procedures have only a limited time for trying IVF with their own eggs and sperm, usually because of the woman's age and her chances of conception. Some people are actually comforted by the limited time they have, because it imposes a boundary for them. They know that they can try IVF for only so long and, if unsuccessful, must then choose a different pathway. Many fertility specialists encourage their patients to think at the outset about the number of IVF cycles they would like to attempt. People can always change their minds, but it often helps to have a goal of trying to conceive with, say, three cycles and then stopping to consider what to do next. Of course, many people are limited to a specific number of cycles by finances, which are discussed further in chapter 16.

After an unsuccessful IVF cycle, the fertility specialist will evaluate the woman or couple to determine if they can proceed directly to another cycle, if they should wait for a while, or if they should consider changes to their treatment plan. As with hormone stimulation, most centers recommend letting the body rest for at least a short time between IVF attempts. Also, not all fertility centers offer cycles every month (they literally don't do any procedures in some months).

Looking at statistics from a 2004 survey of fertility centers, shown in table 14.1, it is possible to get an idea of a woman's chances of having a baby from an IVF cycle using her own eggs. For example, let's consider a woman who is thirty-two years old. She has a 37 percent chance of conceiving and having a baby with any given cycle that she tries; her chance is 37 percent on her first attempt, 37 percent on her second attempt, and so on. But, if we

Table 14.1. Probability of Live Birth with Multiple Cycles of In Vitro Fertilization (from nondonor eggs)

Maternal age in years	One cycle	Two cycles	Three cycles
<35	1/2.7	1/1.7	1/1.3
	(36.9%)	(60.2%)	(74.9%)
35–37	1/3.4	1/2	1/1.5
	(29.3%)	(50%)	(64.7%)
38–40	1/5.1	1/2.8	1/2.1
	(19.5%)	(35.2%)	(47.8%)
41–42	1/9.3	1/4.9	1/3.4
	(10.7%)	(20.3%)	(28.8%)

Source: Society for Assisted Reproductive Technology data. Centers for Disease Control and Prevention. 2004 Assisted Reproductive Technology (ART) Report: National Summary (http://apps.nccd.cdc.gov/ART2004/nation04.asp).

look at a set of three cycles, her chances are greater over all of the cycles combined. So, if this woman decides that she can afford to try up to three IVF cycles, she has a 75 percent chance of conceiving and having a baby from those attempts. In other words, if 100 thirty-two-year-old women commit to trying IVF up to three times in one year, 75 of them will become pregnant during that year and carry the pregnancy to term, some of them on their first attempt, some on their second, and some on their third. Again, as a woman ages, her chances of conceiving and carrying a pregnancy through to a live birth decrease. A forty-two-year-old woman has a 29 percent chance of having a baby with three IVF attempts.

Using Donor Sperm, Eggs, or Embryos

People who decide to use donor eggs or embryos through a fertility center are usually placed on a waiting list, and it may take up to a year, or even longer, to get a donor. If a donor cycle is unsuccessful, the fertility center usually places the woman or couple back on the waiting list for another donor. However, when extra embryos are available in a particular cycle, they can be frozen for the same couple to try another transfer if the initial attempt is unsuccessful. People who choose to find their egg donor on the internet can often decrease their waiting time.

Using donor eggs means three people are involved in the treatment, so the coordination becomes a little more complex. Coordinating three schedules means the wait between cycles may be longer than when a woman uses her own eggs, but the chances of successfully conceiving and carrying the pregnancy to term are higher. Because the maternal age (the donor) is under thirty-five years, the chance for success is 50.5 percent (1 in 2) per cycle. Women who commit to two donor cycles have a 75.5 percent chance of having a baby, and with three cycles, 87.9 percent.

Using donor sperm is much less complicated than using donor eggs. Donor sperm should be immediately available from sperm banks or fertility centers, and an attempt at pregnancy can be made every month. With no maternal fertility problems, including maternal age, the probability of conception with frozen (thawed) donor sperm ranges between 5 and 19 percent. The more insemination cycles attempted, the greater the chances of becoming pregnant, as shown in table 14.2. Women who don't become pregnant after several donor sperm cycles usually change donors, if there is no maternal reason for difficulty conceiving.

Table 14.2. Probability of Conception with Multiple Insemination Cycles

One cycle	Three cycles	Six cycles
1/20 to 1/5.2	1/7 to 1/2.1	1/3.8 to 1/1.4
(5.0% to 19.2%)	(14.3% to 46.9%)	(26.5% to 71.8%)

Note: These data assume there are no maternal fertility problems, including advanced maternal age.

HOW LONG DOES IT TAKE TO FIND A SURROGATE?

The length of time to find a surrogate depends on whether the search is done independently or through an agency. Finding a surrogate independently may be very quick, especially if the surrogate is a relative, or it may take several months if the couple is advertising. Going through an agency requires time for the introductory consultation, drafting a retainer agreement once the individual or couple decides to pursue surrogacy with the agency, submitting a profile (which includes psychological testing), the matching process, and medical evaluation of the surrogate.

When an individual or couple decides to contact an agency about surrogacy, they can usually get a first appointment quickly, within one or two weeks. The initial consultation, drafting the retainer agreement, and submitting a profile takes, on average, two to four weeks. The length of time to match the prospective parents with a surrogate is difficult to predict, because it varies widely depending on the circumstances. Larger agencies (ones that provide all related services such as legal counsel and psychological evaluation) can accomplish matches relatively quickly—generally in one to three months—but it can take longer if few surrogates are available at the time or if the prospective parents have stringent criteria for a surrogate. The more restrictive the criteria, such as wanting a surrogate of a certain race or religion, the longer the wait. Many agencies tell prospective parents that they can expect a wait of six to eight months before a match is made, but many matches are made within a much shorter time. An appropriate match is key to a successful surrogacy arrangement, so this part of the process shouldn't be rushed.

Once matched, the prospective parents meet the surrogate, with the agency acting as the third party to facilitate questions and discussion. Both parties must agree to enter into a contract for the process to continue. If they don't, the prospective parents are typically placed back in the pool to wait for another match (again taking up to six to eight months). If the prospective parents and the surrogate do agree to work together, the agency draws up a contract, which may take up to three months to complete, depending on the agency, the availability of a lawyer, and the information needed. The information required for the contract can include the results of psychological and medical screenings, details of the payment schedule, details about how many IVF procedures will be attempted and how many embryos transferred, and decisions about options in various situations (for example, selective reduction, genetic testing, and drug testing). Once the contract is in place, a trust or escrow account is set up; the prospective parents deposit money into the account and the agency facilitates payment of the surrogate's bills. Setting up the account usually takes no more than a week. If the surrogate doesn't have a health plan, the prospective parents are responsible for finding one for her. It is not uncommon for health plans to have a waiting period before maternity coverage can be used; three months is common.

HOW LONG DOES IT TAKE TO COMPLETE
AN ADOPTION HOME STUDY?

Anyone who wants to adopt, no matter what type of adoption interests them, must undergo a home study. A home study is one of the first steps in the adoption process and usually takes 10 to 20 weeks to complete. The social worker's first appointment with the applicants is usually 6 to 8 weeks after they submit their application to the adoption agency, and it takes the social worker 4 to 12 weeks to write up the home study. The length of time also depends on how quickly the applicants collect the supporting documents. In some areas, the home study may take longer than 20 weeks, especially if there are only a few licensed agencies in the state and they have many applicants.

HOW LONG DOES IT TAKE TO BRING
AN ADOPTED CHILD HOME?

The time it takes from application to bringing an adopted baby or child home depends largely on the type of adoption pursued.

Table 14.3. How Money Spent on Advertising Affects the Chance of Adopting and the Waiting Time to Adoption

Average amount spent on advertising	Percentage of families who successfully adopt	Average waiting time from start of advertising to child placement
$2,000	20	>5 years
$4,000	50	3–5 years
$6,000	80	1–3 years
$8,000	90–95	3–18 months
$10,000	95–100	3–12 months

Source: American Adoptions. Adoption—How Long Is the Wait? (www.americanadoptions .com/adopt/how_long).

With a domestic public agency adoption, people who want to adopt an infant will wait a very long time. Adopting a healthy Caucasian infant, which may not even be an option because of agency restrictions, can take as long as seven to nine years. The wait is shorter—often only 6 to 12 months—to adopt a child of another ethnic background, a child with special needs, or a child older than one year. The usual time with a domestic private agency adoption is 9 to 24 months, although most people have a child within 18 months.

Independent domestic adoptions are generally faster than agency adoptions, taking months instead of years. Most people will bring a baby home within 12 months of beginning the adoption process. The prospective parents' aggressiveness in advertising, which depends on how much they can afford to spend and where they advertise, influences how long it takes to find a birth mother, as shown in table 14.3.

International adoptions are usually completed within one year from the initial application, but the time can vary by country. For example, adoptions from Russia and Ukraine are often completed in under a year, but adoptions from China often take longer than a year due to the popularity of adoptions from this country. After the home study has been completed, the prospective parents must file paperwork with the Immigration and Naturalization Service (INS), and the INS may take two to four months to approve the adoption. Language barriers sometimes lead to communication failures and delays, and unexpected turmoil in a country can also prolong the waiting time.

HOW MUCH TIME WILL YOU NEED
TO TAKE OFF WORK?

Regardless of the pathway you choose, you will almost certainly have to take some time off work. With fertility assistance procedures, such as a hormone stimulation cycle or an IVF cycle, timing is key. For example, hormones usually need to be administered at a specific time during the day (or night), especially the hormones to trigger ovulation. Blood tests and ultrasounds may be required first thing in the morning or at another specific time. An IUI or an egg retrieval is usually scheduled for a particular time, so the timing for the man to provide his sperm sample is critical, often with a window of only one or two hours. Basically, the treatment schedule dictates the couple's—particularly the woman's—daily schedule. It's also worth keeping in mind that some women experience significant side effects with hormone treatments, and as a result they may have difficulty working. People who need to travel from their hometown to a fertility center will be away from work for several days while they undergo a single treatment cycle. Travel is discussed in chapter 15.

A woman who becomes pregnant with fertility assistance may need to reduce her hours at work or even go on bed rest. A recommendation to go on bed rest is probable for a woman pregnant with multiples (and the chance of having multiples is relatively high with fertility assistance). Mothers of twins, triplets, and higher-order multiples average 4, 6, and 12 or more weeks of bed rest, respectively.

Prospective parents who work with a surrogate, if she lives nearby, often want to go to doctors' appointments with her. The surrogate may also need assistance, particularly if she is pregnant with multiples and on bed rest. When a surrogate lives in another state, the intended parents may need to travel to her state during the pregnancy.

Many public agency adoptions require or expect the adoptive parents to attend several hours of preadoption seminars. The adoptive parents may also need to learn about the kinds of problems children may have as a result of experiencing suboptimal environments in their early childhood. When a domestic private or independent adoption is done in another state, the adoptive parents have to travel to the state in which the child is born. They must stay there for 3 to 10 days during the court process and while the state paperwork is filed. To transport the baby from one state to another, an Interstate Compact (a contract between two states) must be signed by the compact administrators in both the sending state (where the baby is born) and the receiving state (where the adoptive parents live). Completing the Interstate Compact usually takes 5 to 7 days, but in some states it takes longer.

For an international adoption, at least one of the adoptive parents has to travel to the child's birth country (some countries may specify that both parents must travel). In some instances, it may be possible for an escort to travel to the child on behalf of the parents. Countries generally require a two- to four-week stay while the adoption is being processed, although the exact length of time varies by country and sometimes adoptive parent may have to stay for several months. In addition, some countries require that one of the adoptive parents stay at home with the child for the first weeks following the adoption.

POSITIVE ASPECTS TO CONSIDER

- Waiting for a baby or child to arrive prolongs the anticipation and gives time to prepare for the new addition to the family.
- Probably the most enjoyable reason to take leave from work is for pregnancy, childbirth, or adoption.

FURTHER READING

L. Beauvais-Godwin and R. Godwin. *Complete Adoption Book: Everything You Need to Know to Adopt a Child*. Adams Media, 2000.

J. N. Erichsen and H. R. Erichsen. *How to Adopt Internationally: A Guide for Agency-Directed and Independent Adoptions*. Mesa House, 2003.

Everything Surrogacy. www.everythingsurrogacy.com.

J. Meyers-Thompson and S. Perkins. *Fertility for Dummies*. Wiley, 2003.

R. Mintzer. *Yes, You Can Adopt! A Comprehensive Guide to Adoption*. Avalon, Carroll and Graf, 2003.

I HAD AN UNSUCCESSFUL MARRIAGE in my twenties and told myself that I wouldn't marry again. I didn't have any children from that marriage, and I was content to live child-free and enjoy my nieces and nephews. And then, when I was forty-three, I met a wonderful man who was 13 years younger than me. We got married. I was still content not to have children, but my husband wanted a child and persuaded me. We tried to get pregnant without success for four months and then went to a fertility specialist. Because of my age, the specialist recommended that we not waste our time with artificial insemination but go immediately to IVF. I think we were very, very fortunate, because I became pregnant from our first IVF cycle. The pregnancy turned out to be twins, which was daunting news to receive. My husband was elated, and I slowly became more excited as I got used to the idea. I didn't have a great time during the pregnancy; I had high blood pressure and at 26 weeks I was put on bed rest. It was hard to suddenly be so dependent and to be so immobile, but I knew I had to do it for the sake of the babies. I made it to 36 weeks, which I'm told is pretty good for twins, and then my blood pressure started causing more problems. My babies, nonidentical boys, were born by Cesarean section.

It's amazing that I spent so much of my life without children, because I now can't imagine life without them. My two sons are now five years old, and though I'm often utterly exhausted by the end of the day, I can't think of another life I'd rather have.

Chapter 15

HASSLE COSTS

Travel, Appointments, Forms, and Documents

Every option for becoming a parent involves some degree of hassle, including paperwork, travel, appointments, court dates, and so on. The time costs described in the previous chapter are intertwined with the hassles, and it inevitably takes time to deal with these.

FERTILITY ASSISTANCE

The Possibility of Travel

Most metropolitan areas in the United States have an assisted reproductive technology (ART) clinic and large cities have several, particularly in the Northeast. However, people living in smaller towns or rural areas may be a long way from the nearest clinic, and some states don't have any ART clinics at all. For example, residents of Alaska have very few local options and may decide to travel hundreds of miles for assistance at a fertility clinic. People who travel away from their hometown for fertility assistance should plan to be away for about five to seven days for a hormone stimulation cycle and about two weeks for an in vitro fertilization (IVF) cycle. If a woman has already been through at least one cycle, some centers may allow her to begin the hormone injections for subsequent attempts at home, with monitoring at a local facility. Doing so will minimize the length of time the woman has to be away from home. In 2004, 411 ART clinics submitted data to the Society for Assisted Reproductive Technology; these clinics and their locations are shown on the SART website (www .sart.org).

Centers that offer donor egg or embryo services are even more scarce than IVF centers. However, people who decide to use donor egg or embryo services in a state other than their state of residence may only need to make two visits: the first visit for the initial evaluation, and the second for the embryo transfer. Any additional testing needed before the embryo transfer, as well as the follow-up pregnancy testing, can be performed by a fertility center in their home state. Being a donor egg or embryo recipient is relatively easy and involves fewer clinic visits than undergoing an IVF procedure. The donor, not the recipient, is the person who receives the frequent monitoring and hormone injections prior to embryo transfer.

Surrogacy is not legal in every state, so people interested in working with a surrogate may have to find one in another state. They will then have to travel to the surrogate's state at least twice—once to meet the surrogate before entering an agreement and once when the baby is born—although many prospective parents will make more than these two visits during the prenatal period. If the male partner of a couple is contributing the sperm in a traditional surrogacy arrangement, he will need to travel an additional time to provide the sample. For a gestational surrogacy, both the woman and man providing the eggs and sperm will need to travel to the surrogate's state for the egg retrieval, to provide the sperm sample, and possibly for the embryo transfer, depending on the wait between fertilization and transfer (most intended parents want to stay for the transfer anyway). Alternatively, the intended parents in either traditional or gestational arrangements may provide transportation for the surrogate to come to their state of residence for the insemination, egg retrieval, embryo transfer, and any other necessary procedures. In many gestational surrogacy arrangements, both the intended mother (who will provide her own eggs) and the surrogate (who must prepare her uterus) undergo IVF medication and monitoring in their own states, with communication and collaboration between their local fertility clinics. If the surrogate's nearest fertility clinic is out of town, the intended parents are responsible for her travel expenses to and from the clinic (in addition to her medication and clinic fees, child care, time off work, and any other expenses).

Paperwork and Documents

All fertility centers require that consent forms be signed for early fertility assistance or ART treatment. These consent forms are signed before the treatment begins, but occasionally it's also necessary to sign some forms on the day of the egg retrieval. The center may ask whether it has permission to use sperm, eggs, embryos, or any other tissue for research. The woman or couple receiving the treatment also need to decide if they will freeze any extra embryos that aren't transferred. As discussed in chapter 3, people who choose not to freeze extra embryos must decide what's to be done with them, such as donating them to another couple or terminating them in an appropriate manner.

Surrogacy arrangements require a variety of paperwork. When working with an agency, the individual or couple must write a "Dear Surrogate" letter, which is a personal statement about what they want from a surrogacy arrangement. The agency uses this letter to make a match with a surrogate. People who independently seek a surrogate also need to write a personal statement about the arrangement they want, to be read by possible applicants, and they then need to review the applications they receive. The "Dear Surrogate" letter should address a range of issues, including:

- The type of surrogacy (traditional or gestational)
- The desired time frame for starting and completing the surrogacy
- Their family's feelings about surrogacy
- Their feelings about abortion, selective reduction, and multiple births

- The number of cycles they would like to attempt
- The coverage of the surrogate's fees and expenses, including both medical and life insurance
- The amount of contact desired

Once a match is made with a surrogate, whether traditional or gestational, the individual or couple need to enter into a contractual agreement with the surrogate. When working through an agency, the agency facilitates drawing up the contract with a lawyer. As described in chapter 14, a variety of information must be included in the contract, including psychological and medical test results, information about payment, and details of the procedures to be undertaken in achieving and monitoring the pregnancy. In an independent arrangement, the individual or couple seeking the surrogacy must find and work with an attorney to draft the document. In either case, court visits will probably also be necessary.

DOMESTIC ADOPTIONS

The Home Study

All domestic adoptions require a home study. It may also become necessary for anyone interested in being the recipient of a donated embryo to have a home study; in a few states, a home study is already a requirement for recipients of donor embryos. The social worker who conducts the home study will want to see a variety of documents from the applicants. Most documents need to be either originals or notarized copies of originals. People who provide a document or letter of reference for the applicants may have to sign it in the presence of a notary. The documents required in most home studies include the following:

- Birth certificate for each applicant
- Marriage license
- Divorce decree (if applicable)
- Medical report on each applicant's health
- Income verification (W-2s, copies of income tax returns, pay stubs)

- Financial statements
- Personal reference letters from friends (three to five)
- Child abuse/FBI clearance (usually, fingerprints are required from either a police precinct or a Family Court)
- Insurance verification for both health and life insurance
- An autobiographical statement from each prospective parent

Most home studies require a personal interview, and generally there is more than one interview. At least one interview takes place in the applicants' home, and during the meeting, the social worker also looks at the home itself to be sure it is safe and childproof. Applicants who have pets, guns, medications, chemicals, or a swimming pool must establish proper safety procedures to satisfy the requirements of their state or, in the case of international adoptions, of the child's birth country.

The Portfolio for Independent Adoptions

People who decide to adopt independently should prepare a portfolio that reflects what they can offer as parents. The portfolio is the adoptive parents' advertising tool, and its preparation takes thoughtful consideration about what to include. The portfolio generally includes biographical information, photographs, a letter to the birth mother, and possibly the report of the home study. The adoptive parents also need to find a lawyer and determine how they will advertise for birth mothers. A lawyer can often give advice about the best advertising tactics.

Finalizing a Domestic Adoption

After the initial placement of a child, postplacement visits will take place for the next two to six months. Assuming all goes well with the postplacement visits and the birth mother has signed a waiver of parental rights, the adoptive parents will have one last court date to finalize the adoption. The judge, lawyer, adoptive parents, and sometimes the social worker are present for this court visit, which usually takes only about 15 minutes. The adoptive parents are asked to take the stand and must state facts such as their marriage date, the child's birth date, and the child's placement date. The judge asks questions to be sure the parents know the legal implications of accepting the child for adoption. The judge then formally signs the adoption decree to finalize the adoption.

INTERNATIONAL ADOPTIONS

International adoptions obviously include overseas travel, which requires a passport and often other documentation. In addition, international adoptions require many more documents and forms than domestic adoptions. They also involve other hassles—namely, those associated with dealing with another language. Applicants must rely on the agency and its interpreters for much of the information they receive about their child, and all of the documents must be translated. Depending on the country, adoptive parents may need to have the notary public's signature certified and verified by the secretary of state in the state where their documents were notarized.

The international adoption process is not as onerous as it may at first seem from the following descriptions of the additional hassles and paperwork. Adoption agencies are there to help their clients determine what they need to do and where they have to send the various documents and forms that they gather.

The Home Study

The home study for an international adoption proceeds much like the home study for a domestic adoption, and it can be completed even before the applicants have decided which country they would like to adopt from. The documents required for the home study in an international adoption generally include the following:

- Certified birth certificates for each family member
- Certified marriage license
- Certified death certificates for former spouses, if applicable
- Divorce decree, if applicable

- Letter from each applicant's employer stating length of employment and annual salary
- Statement of net worth, written by applicants or their accountant
- Copies of each applicant's health and life insurance policies
- Medical examination forms signed by a physician for each family member; these forms are generally considered current for one year
- Photocopies of each applicant's federal income tax returns for the last three years; the applicant needs to write "I certify that this is a true copy of the original" and then sign and date the statement in the presence of a notary
- For each family member over age eighteen, a letter from the local police department stating that the individual has no criminal record; some countries also require a state police clearance
- Reference letters from at least three people not related to the applicants; ideally, the letters should come from professionals or leaders in the community, such as the applicant's physician, lawyer, or clergy person, and they need to be signed by a notary, the secretary of state, and the foreign consul
- Child abuse clearances and criminal clearances for each member of the family over eighteen (from the state's social services department)
- Three sets of photographs of the applicants and their children, if applicable, in front of their home, and three sets of individual close-ups

The Foreign Dossier

Once the applicants decide on a country, the agency works with them to prepare a foreign dossier. Although the task may seem formidable, most of the documents required for the foreign dossier are the same as those already collected for the home study. In addition, the foreign dossier usually must include the following:

- The application form of the overseas child-placing agency or entity (government authorities in charge of adoption in many countries have their own application forms)
- A letter to the overseas child-placing agency or entity (this letter may be written by the agency that the applicants are working with)
- A copy of the home study report
- The agency's license
- A photocopy of form I-600A or I-600 (described below)
- The INS's approval to adopt (form I-171H)
- The international processing contract (a document that explains the agency's and applicants' responsibilities in locating a child and arranging legal custody of the child)
- Photocopies of the first two pages of each applicant's passport

INS Forms

The INS requires prospective parents to fill out several forms: I-600A and/or I-600 and I-171H.

Form I-600A (Application for Advance Processing of Orphan Petition) is usually the first to be filled out and is used when a child has not yet been identified. Once a child is identified and assigned to the prospective parents, form I-600 (Petition to Classify Orphan as an Immediate Relative) must be completed. The advantage of sending in form I-600A first is that it expedites the adoption process. I-600A is not compulsory, but I-600 is.

The purpose of form I-600 is to verify that the child to be adopted is truly an orphan. The I-600 form must be accompanied by several documents that verify the child's status as an orphan. These documents can include the following, depending on the country:

- Proof of the orphan's age
- Death certificate(s) of the orphan's parents, if applicable
- Proof that the child has been lawfully adopted abroad, or, if the child is to be adopted in the United States, evidence that

any preadoption requirements of the state of the orphan's proposed residence have been met
- Proof that the orphan's only surviving parent, if there is one,
  cannot care for the child and has, in writing, forever and irrev-
  ocably released the orphan for emigration and adoption
- Proof that the orphan has been unconditionally abandoned
  to an orphanage, if that is the case

When the INS receives either I-600 or I-600A, it then sends
the applicants form I-171H (Notice of Favorable Determination
Concerning Application for Advance Processing of Orphan Petition). I-171H indicates that once a child has been assigned to
prospective parents, they can proceed with the adoption.

Applicants also need to get fingerprinted by the FBI for INS
requirements.

Bringing an Adopted Child Home

Once in the child's birth country, the adoptive parents need to take
their child for a medical clearance examination. The embassy or
consulate identifies a specific clinic to take the child to, and although the exam is generally quick, the visit to the clinic can be
a whole-day affair. The adoptive parents must also fill out a visa
application and will need to get a passport for their child, which
the agency may take care of. The adoptive parents must go for an
interview at the embassy or consulate before the child's visa is
issued. Documents needed for the child's visa include:

- The visa application
- Photographs of the child for the visa
- The child's birth certificate
- The country's adoption decree of guardianship (must be trans-
  lated into English)
- The child's passport
- The child's medical evaluation

When the adopted child has entered the United States, the
adoptive parents may need to readopt the child. Whether or not

it's necessary to readopt in the United States depends on the child's visa. An IR-4 visa indicates either that the adoptive parents were given guardianship but did not legally adopt the child in his or her birth country or that the adoptive parents did not see the child before he or she was adopted. In the case of a child having an IR-4 visa, federal law requires the adoptive parents to adopt or readopt the child in the United States. An IR-3 visa indicates that the child was legally adopted by the adoptive parents in his or her country of birth. In this instance, the adoptive parents may not be required to readopt, but it is still advisable to do so.

Readoption is a simple and inexpensive process. The adoptive parents need to show copies of the home study, the child's birth certificate, documents indicating parental abandonment or relinquishment, and the adoption decree from the foreign country. Some states may also ask for documentation of postplacement visits. Once all the paperwork has been filed, the adoptive parents will go to court for the child's final adoption.

Once a child with an IR-4 visa has been readopted, the adoptive parents can apply for the child's citizenship in the United States with INS form N-643 (Certificate of Citizenship on Behalf of an Adopted Child). A child who received an IR-3 visa is eligible for automatic citizenship in the United States. However, parents must still file form N-643. Documents that must accompany N-643 include:

- The child's alien registration card
- The child's birth certificate
- The final adoption decree
- Evidence that at least one of the adoptive parents is a U.S. citizen
- The adoptive parents' marriage certificate or divorce decree (if divorced), or the death certificate of the spouse if a parent is widowed
- Recent passport photographs of the child

POSITIVE ASPECTS TO CONSIDER

- Traveling for any of the pathways to parenthood gives you a good excuse to visit a place you want to explore.
- After going through the adoption process, you will have all of your important documents available and organized for any future needs.

FURTHER READING

C. Adamec. *The Complete Idiot's Guide to Adoption*. Alpha Books, 1998.

J. N. Erichsen and H. R. Erichsen. *How to Adopt Internationally: A Guide for Agency-Directed and Independent Adoptions*. Mesa House, 2003.

R. Mintzer. *Yes, You Can Adopt! A Comprehensive Guide to Adoption*. Avalon, Carroll and Graf, 2003.

R. O. Sweet and P. Bryan. *Adopt International: Everything You Need to Know to Adopt a Child from Abroad*. Noonday Press, 1996.

● ───

I WENT THROUGH EARLY MENOPAUSE in my late twenties, so when my husband and I got married several years later we already knew that we'd have to consider other ways of having children. Our choices were using eggs donated by another woman or adopting. Because we were both still quite young and healthy, we decided to try donor eggs using my husband's sperm. I also really wanted to experience pregnancy.

I wanted a donor who had my characteristics—olive skin, dark hair and eyes. We went on a list at a fertility center and were lucky to get a donor match just two months later. We didn't meet the donor, but we agreed through the fertility center that we'd have two attempts—if the first attempt didn't take, we'd try a second time and the donor would go through stimulation again to provide fresh eggs. We were so excited to start the procedure and had high hopes. The donor produced only five eggs, but we ended up with two good-quality embryos and both were transferred. I didn't become pregnant, though.

We took a break, and four months later, on the second attempt, we again transferred two embryos and one of them took. We were ecstatic, but our joy was short-lived—I miscarried at 5 weeks. Our egg donor wasn't ready to go through the stimulation again, so we had to decide whether we'd wait for another donor or proceed with adoption. That's when a friend told us about overseas clinics. My husband and I are lucky that we both have good jobs and could even consider the expensive proposition of going overseas. We spent some time researching different countries and clinics, and we decided on one in Spain. We agreed between us that we'd make the trip a holiday, and we'd only go once. If that attempt didn't work, we'd adopt.

The procedure was basically the same as we'd gone through at home, but for us there was one important difference: I became pregnant and the pregnancy took! Our son was born last year, and everyone remarks on how much he looks like me. This makes me so happy! When our son was born we thought we'd be content with one child, but we've enjoyed him so much that we're now thinking of trying again for a second child.

—— ●

Chapter 16

FINANCIAL COSTS

Which Options Are Affordable?

Financial costs are more objective than some of the other costs described in this book, because they can be clearly measured and information about these costs is readily available from various resources. However, they may vary from clinic to clinic and from agency to agency, and they are also likely to change over time. The information in this chapter will nevertheless provide you with a good approximation of what costs to expect in the United States from each of the options for becoming a parent.

FERTILITY ASSISTANCE

Fertility assistance costs range from a few hundred to several thousand dollars, as shown in table 16.1. Compared with early assistance techniques, the cost rises dramatically for assisted reproductive technology (ART) procedures. One in vitro fertilization (IVF) cycle can cost $9,500 to $16,500, and using intracytoplasmic sperm injection (ICSI) in conjunction with IVF costs about another $1,500. Although ICSI cycles cost more, the probability of success is higher. The IVF cost includes ultrasounds, lab fees, anesthesia, egg retrieval, embryo transfer, and professional and technical fees. Medications are extra and usually cost an additional $2,000 per cycle, with variability from woman to woman. Older

Table 16.1. General Range of Costs for Fertility Assistance

Tests and procedures	General cost
Sperm analysis	$100–$150
Hysterosalpingogram	$1,200–$1,700
Laparoscopy	$3,000–$10,000
Early fertility assistance techniques	
• Intrauterine sperm insemination	$150–$700
• Intracervical sperm insemination	$100–$700
• Hormone stimulation[1]	
Oral (Clomid)	$1,500–$1,900/cycle
Injectable medications[2]	$2,500–$2,700/cycle
Assisted reproductive technology	
• IVF alone[2]	$9,500–$16,500/cycle
• IVF with intracytoplasmic sperm injection[2]	$11,000–$18,000/cycle
• Preimplantation genetic diagnosis	$4,000–$5,000

Source: Websites for various fertility centers (accessed in 2007).

1. Cost includes medication, ultrasound monitoring, and blood tests for hormone levels.

2. Cost is higher for older women who need higher medication doses for stimulation. The rest of the in vitro fertilization (IVF) cost is fixed.

women, in particular, usually require more hormones to achieve the desired stimulation response, so their medication costs will be higher, sometimes hundreds of dollars more per cycle. Preimplantation genetic diagnosis (PGD) is particularly expensive, costing around $4,000 to $5,000. In addition to the procedures, there are other expenses to take into account, including lost wages, travel, and accommodation.

The cost varies by fertility center, with factors such as geographic location influencing the total cost of fertility assistance procedures. It may be possible to receive a discount for certain tests or procedures. For example, some centers give a discounted rate for people who commit up-front to two or three cycles. The details depend on the agency, but in some instances people don't get any money back if they successfully conceive on the first cycle. Other centers offer a refund to people who don't successfully conceive after two or three cycles, although the up-front fee is higher for refund programs.

Costs are higher in the United States than in some other countries. Some people opt to go overseas where the medical costs can be much lower. A small number of Americans have sought fertility assistance procedures in, for example, South Africa, Israel, Italy, Germany, and Canada.

As described in previous chapters, ART procedures increase the chance of a multiple pregnancy. For people who have limited resources and wish for more than one child, this higher chance may be an attractive aspect of fertility assistance options. However, a mother will probably need more help with multiples when they are born, which is an immediate added expense following pregnancy. The likelihood of being put on bed rest during a pregnancy with multiples is also higher than for a singleton pregnancy, so a woman carrying multiples will probably have to take time off work during her pregnancy.

Donor Sperm

There are a few things to consider when buying donor sperm. The sperm can be inserted with either an intracervical (ICI) or an intrauterine (IUI) procedure, and the procedure affects the cost. Sperm prepared for ICI are less expensive than sperm prepared for IUI, and the ICI procedure itself is less expensive. However, IUI has a higher success rate, so fewer attempts are usually needed to conceive when using IUI. IUI-ready sperm are available from sperm banks and cost more than sperm that haven't been prepared, but it won't be necessary to pay for sperm processing at the fertility center.

Some sperm banks include other options for the sperm they sell. For example, they may specify whether the sperm are from doctorate donors (men who have acquired or are in school working toward a doctorate degree) versus nondoctorate donors. Sperm samples from doctorate donors cost more.

The cost for a sperm sample plus an insemination is generally between $200 and $700, including shipping costs. The shipping will be more expensive if the sperm are needed on a weekend or are shipped internationally.

The insemination procedure must be done when the woman is ovulating, so most fertility specialists recommend two inseminations spaced one day apart. In this case, it's necessary to order two vials of sperm (at double the cost). Some people choose to order more vials to ensure future access to sperm from the same donor.

A woman is more likely to achieve pregnancy with fresh sperm, so fewer cycles are needed to become pregnant. Therefore, if fresh sperm are used, the overall cost of achieving a successful pregnancy is lower than when frozen sperm are used. Using fresh sperm is generally only an option for women whose male partner is providing the sperm or for women who otherwise know their sperm donor.

Donor Eggs

In the United States, the cost of using donor eggs varies greatly from clinic to clinic. People pursuing this option can expect to pay between $15,000 and $25,000 for one IVF cycle with donor eggs. The cost includes compensation for the donor (usually about $5,000), one cycle of IVF (usually $9,500 to $16,500), and possibly legal fees (about $600 to $1,500). As with using one's own eggs, cycles using ICSI are more expensive, by about $1,500. Agency fees are in addition to these costs and may be as high as $8,000.

People who want a donor with very specific characteristics should be prepared to pay even more. For example, female students at Stanford have in the past asked for $50,000 in compensation for egg donation. People whose insurance policy does not cover donor egg treatment may have to pay the entire cost up-front.

Donor Embryos

A couple who uses donor embryos can expect to pay $2,500 to $5,000 for a single cycle. This cost may include a home study (if required by the state), fertility center fees, specific testing and screening expenses (including screening for sexually transmitted diseases), and expenses incurred in storing embryos or transferring them to the clinic. Several items are not included in this cost estimate, including medications, counseling, and legal fees. One of the most variable costs from state to state is the home study, which can cost from $500 to $3,000. The donor couple receives no financial compensation, but the recipient couple reimburses the donors for any costs associated with the embryo donation process.

Fertility Assistance Insurance

Health insurance plans may or may not cover fertility assistance services, depending on where you live and the type of insurance plan you have. Many health insurance plans don't routinely cover fertility treatments, because infertility isn't regarded as a legitimate medical condition. As of December 2007, 14 states had laws that require insurers to either cover or offer some coverage for an infertility diagnosis and treatment. Those states are Arkansas, California, Connecticut, Hawaii, Illinois, Maryland, Massachusetts, Montana, New Jersey, New York, Ohio, Rhode Island, Texas, and West Virginia. In the remaining states, many insurance plans offer no coverage or cover only the basic workup.

SURROGACY

Surrogacy arrangements can cost relatively little if a family member or friend acts as the surrogate and doesn't expect payment. In this case, medical and legal costs would be the only expenses. However, most people have to hire a surrogate. The cost of using a surrogate, whether gestational or traditional, varies, depending on how the arrangement is set up and what's included. Gestational surrogacy is more expensive than traditional surrogacy, given the medical costs involved with IVF (gestational) versus insemination (traditional). A contract arranged through an agency typically

Table 16.2. General Costs of Using an Agency for Selected Surrogacy Services

Service	Average range of cost
Agency fee for the surrogacy arrangement	$6,000–$16,000
Agency fee for arranging egg donation	$2,000–$6,000
Surrogate's compensation	$10,000–$40,000
Egg donor's compensation	$2,000–$10,000
Surrogate's legal counsel fees	$300–$1,500
Surrogate's health insurance (if she has none)	$125–$250/month
Surrogate's psychological counseling	$500–$700
Surrogate's parental relinquishment (if needed)	$250–$750

Sources: everythingsurrogacy.com (www.everythingsurrogacy.com); TASC: The American Surrogacy Center (www.surrogacy.com); T. M. Erickson and M. Lathus. *Assisted Reproduction: The Complete Guide to Having a Baby with the Help of a Third Party.* iUniverse, 2005.

totals $22,000 to $120,000. The cost range for a selection of possible surrogacy services obtained through an agency is shown in table 16.2. The majority of the costs come from the medical, legal, and agency (if applicable) fees and the surrogate compensation. Possible additional expenses include lost wages, child care, housekeeping, and travel.

Surrogate compensation can depend on the woman's experience as a surrogate in the past. According to Stacy Ziegler in *Pathways to Parenthood: The Ultimate Guide to Surrogacy*, the average compensation for a first-time surrogate is between $16,000 and $23,000, while the fee for a proven surrogate can range anywhere from $20,000 to $40,000. These amounts are solely for surrogate compensation and don't include the cost of medications to prepare the surrogate for embryo transfer or insemination or the cost of the surrogate's prenatal care and delivery (if they aren't covered by her insurance). Any medical expenses that aren't covered by an insurance plan are paid by the intended parents. In addition, all parties to a surrogacy arrangement are encouraged to receive counseling, which would also be paid for by the intended parents.

The surrogate's compensation includes living costs (partial reimbursement of rent or mortgage and partial payment for food and clothing), travel costs, lost wages (if applicable), disability/life insurance coverage, and other related expenses that are allocated within a surrogacy agreement. The exact breakdown of allowable expenses varies according to state law, and reimbursement for expenses that would have occurred regardless of pregnancy is not allowed. Compensation payments begin once pregnancy is confirmed, and continue throughout the pregnancy and for a specified postpartum period. Typically, surrogacy contracts are set up so that the intended parents make monthly payments to the surrogate mother for a fixed period of time.

The legal fees to draft the surrogacy contract are typically $1,000 to $1,500, and the legal fees for amending the birth certificate average between $750 and $1,000. These costs don't include legal representation for the surrogate, who is sometimes advised to hire her own lawyer.

The surrogacy contract should designate the formation of an escrow account or trust fund, which may be established and held by an attorney, a bank, or an escrow office. This account should have sufficient funds to pay medical fees, insurance premiums, the surrogate's expenses, attorneys' and other professionals' fees, and other expenses. Generally, the intended parents deposit a lump sum of at least $30,000 into this account and they receive a monthly statement of debits.

ADOPTION

General Expenses

All adoptions include certain expenses, such as the cost of a home study. Other expenses depend on the type of adoption pursued. The items that prospective parents must be prepared to pay for with each type of adoption are listed in table 16.3, and a summary of total costs is in table 16.4. The following sections provide details about the cost breakdown for each type of adoption.

Table 16.3. Expenses Associated with Each Type of Adoption

	Domestic public agency	Domestic private agency	Domestic independent	International
Home study	X	X	X	X
Advertising			X	
Agency administrative costs	X	X		X
Birth mother's living expenses		X	X	
Birth mother's medical expenses		X	X	
Birth mother's counseling		X	X	
Attorney fees			X	X
Foreign country fees				X

Table 16.4. Summary of Total Adoption Costs for Each Type of Adoption

Domestic public agency	0–$2,500
Domestic private agency	$5,000–$30,000+
Domestic independent	$8,000–$40,000+
International	$7,000–$30,000+

Source: Data from Child Welfare Information Gateway. Available at: adoption.com. Cost of Adopting (http://statistics.adoption.com/information/statistics-on-cost-of-adopting.html).

Domestic Adoptions

The total cost for a domestic adoption varies widely and depends on a variety of factors:

- Type of adoption (public or private agency; independent)
- Where in the United States the adoption occurs
- Whether or not the agency charges a sliding-scale fee based on family income
- The amount of state or federal subsidy available for adoption of a child with special needs

Table 16.5. Costs for Domestic Adoption

Category	Range of costs
Agency fees	
Application fee	$100–$500
Home study and preparation services[1]	$500–$3,000
Postplacement supervision	$200–$1,500
Physical exam (each parent)	$35–$150
Psychiatric evaluations (each parent, if required)	$250–$400
Attorney fees	
Document preparation	$500–$2,000
Petition and court representation	$2,500–$12,000
Advertising (usual range)[2]	$500–$5,000
Birth mother's (parents') expenses[3]	
Obstetrical and perinatal expenses[4]	0–$20,000
Living expenses	$500–$12,000
Legal representation	$500–$1,500
Counseling	$500–$2,000

Source: Data from Child Welfare Information Gateway. Available at: adoption.com. Estimates for Specific Adoption Costs (http://statistics.adoption.com/information/statistics-on-cost-of-adopting.html#estimate).

1. A home study is required for every type of adoption and the cost depends on the state of residence. Although the range is large, the usual cost is between $750 and $1,750. The study costs more if it is an agency-affiliated home study. Private organizations can also be licensed to do home studies. The cost doesn't affect the quality of the home study.

2. See the comments on advertising in the discussion of independent adoptions in the text below.

3. Allowable amount and type of expenses are usually restricted by state law and subject to review by the court.

4. Zero if covered by birth mother's insurance.

- Federal or state tax credits available for reimbursement of adoption expenses
- Employer adoption benefits

Table 16.5 provides an approximate range for the cost of each item involved in a domestic adoption, whether it be an agency-facilitated or an independent adoption.

Domestic Agency Adoptions

Domestic adoptions through public agencies are generally the least expensive of all types of adoption, with up-front fees ranging from nothing to $2,500. State and federal subsidies are often available for adopting children with special needs and, in addition, a special needs child adopted in the United States is probably entitled to health services paid for by Medicaid or other funds. Some people opt to be a foster parent before they adopt; foster parents receive a monthly stipend (usually $300 to $700) for a child's living expenses.

The least expensive private agency adoptions are those done through agencies affiliated with a particular religion. These agencies often do not charge directly for the birth mother's expenses, or they may have a set fee or sliding scale of fees based on the adoptive parents' income. If the birth mother changes her mind, there is no charge. (Birth mothers who go to a religion-affiliated agency are more likely to change their mind.)

Adoptions through other private agencies can be much more expensive. The administrative and personnel costs involved in a private agency adoption can range from $10,000 to $15,000; this cost may not cover the birth mother's medical, living, counseling, legal, and transportation expenses. With some agencies, the adoptive parents pay a birth mother's expenses indirectly as part of the agency's fees, in which case the fee will range from $20,000 to $30,000. Although a domestic private agency adoption may cost as little as $5,000, the average total estimate for a successful adoption through a large agency is $20,000 to $30,000.

Domestic Independent Adoptions

An independent adoption usually costs between $15,000 and $25,000, but it can be as little as $8,000 or as much as $50,000. The variability is related primarily to how the prospective parents find a birth mother and whether they need to cover her medical bills.

Most people find a birth mother by placing advertisements. Advertising costs can range from $100 to $1,500 per week (for example, in *USA Today* or *TV Guide*). Advertising on the internet can range from a $150 donation to thousands of dollars. As mentioned in chapter 14, people who spend more on advertising tend to successfully complete an independent adoption in a relatively short time—months to about a year. By way of comparison, large agencies that advertise for birth mothers usually spend about $8,000 on advertising per successful adoption. The goal of advertising is to find a birth mother, so prospective parents need to provide their contact information in their ads. Although it is an additional expense, many people find it helpful to have a separate "baby" phone line.

A second potentially large cost in an independent adoption is medical coverage for the birth mother. If the birth mother has her own medical insurance or qualifies for Medicaid coverage, then the prospective parents need only pay for the medical expenses of the baby and any counseling requested by the birth mother or birth parents. However, if the birth mother has no insurance, then the prospective parents must cover all medical costs as well. Unfortunately, some birth mothers claim unnecessary or fraudulent expenses, so prospective parents need to be aware of this risk.

It is illegal to buy a baby, so prospective parents can't pay the birth mother for placing her child with them. However, they do pay the birth mother reasonable living expenses, which usually range from $2,000 to $10,000 for the duration of the pregnancy. These funds should be placed in escrow with an attorney for the purpose of paying living expenses. The court reviews all payments made to the birth mother to determine if they are appropriate.

When adopting independently, it's vital that a lawyer be hired to ensure that legal matters are properly addressed. Prospective parents can expect to pay $3,000 to $14,000 for the services of their attorney. The prospective parents also pay the cost of the birth mother's attorney, which usually totals $2,000 to $3,500. If a child is adopted from another state, it's advisable to hire an attorney in both states to ensure that all applicable laws are complied with.

The costs discussed here are for successfully completed adoptions. Sometimes an arrangement with a birth mother falls through, and the prospective parents lose the money they have invested up to that time. It used to be possible to buy adoption cancellation insurance, which offered protection against financial loss if the adoption fell through, but as of January 2008 this insurance is no longer available.

International Adoptions

International adoptions can vary in cost from a few thousand to tens of thousands of dollars. The fees charged by international adoption agencies generally range from $7,000 to $30,000 and include services such as the U.S. State Department visa application, psychological evaluations and physical examinations, transportation, accommodation and meals in the foreign country, the foreign agency placement fee, translation and escort services, passport office fees, and postplacement supervision, among other expenses. Factors that can affect the agency fee include:

- Whether the placement entity in the foreign country is a government agency or a government-subsidized orphanage
- Whether or not the foreign country requires translation or authentication of the dossier documents
- Whether or not a "donation" must be made to the foreign orphanage or agency
- Whether or not the foreign country requires one or both adoptive parents to travel to the country for interviews and court hearings, and how long the adoptive parent or parents must remain in the country

There may also be additional costs not covered in the agency fees, such as:

- Child foster care (usually required in South and Central American adoptions)
- Parents' travel to the country
- Escorting fees, charged when parents do not travel but in-

Table 16.6. Immigration and Naturalization Service (INS) and State Department Fees

Service	Cost
Filing fee for forms I-600A, I-600	$405
Filing fee for form N-643	$125
Immigrant visa application fee	$260
Immigrant visa issuance fee	$60

Source: Data from Child Welfare Information Gateway. Available at: adoption.com. Estimates for Specific Adoption Costs (http://statistics.adoption.com/information/statistics-on-cost-of-adopting.html#estimate).

stead hire escorts to accompany the child on the flight to the United States
- The child's medical care and treatment before the adoption takes place (occasionally required in South and Central America

The INS/State Department charges fees for the services it provides in international adoptions, as shown in table 16.6.

By way of example, in December 2007, the overall average cost to adopt a child from China was estimated at $22,000 and for a child from Russia was $35,000. The overall cost includes agency fees, INS costs, and any extra costs listed above.

Although unusual, it is possible that a licensed agency taking money for an international adoption does not have the contacts or expertise to facilitate a successful adoption. Regrettably, in this circumstance, the adoptive parents lose their money. The risk of this happening is minimal if you use large, well-established agencies. Before you apply through a particular agency, ask to talk to previous clients about their experience.

Some people opt to conduct their own international adoptions—often called parent-initiated, direct, or independent adoptions—because they are less expensive. However, independent adoptions involve some additional risks. One notable risk is that the child selected by the prospective parents may not meet the definition of an orphan and therefore may not be permitted to migrate to the United States.

Adoption Credits and Benefits

The federal tax credit to help defray the costs of domestic and international adoptions expired in 2002, with the exception of domestic adoptions of special needs children. Parents who adopt a child with special needs from within the United States qualify for a $6,000 credit. In addition, children with special needs may qualify for an adoption subsidy, which is paid to adoptive families to help them pay for their child's need for ongoing therapies or treatment. Several states give tax credits for families adopting children through public agencies or the state's child welfare system. Following finalization of a public agency adoption, families can also apply for reimbursement of expenses, up to $2,000, related to the adoption. Both tax credits and tax-free adoption benefits decline as the annual family income increases, and there are no credits or benefits for families above a specific income level.

HIDDEN COSTS

Although this chapter focuses on the immediate costs to achieve parenthood, it's also worth considering some of the costs that will arise once you become a parent. Some of the pathways described in this book have the possibility of causing higher than average costs in the early days of parenthood. For example, parents of multiples may need to consider paying for additional help. Multiples are also more likely than singletons to have medical problems. As described in chapter 12, certain adopted children are at higher risk of specific mental health disorders. Families with children who are difficult to care for sometimes require both counseling and respite care. Medical, mental health, and behavioral issues can necessitate costly and ongoing treatment. You should consider the potential for these unexpected expenses when thinking about the various pathways to parenthood.

POSITIVE ASPECTS TO CONSIDER

- The time involved in pursuing parenthood is limited. Although the bills may seem overwhelming initially, they will not continue forever.
- Some options are financially very reasonable.

FURTHER READING

C. Adamac. *The Complete Idiot's Guide to Adoption.* Alpha Books, 1998.

Adoption.com. The Costs of Adopting: A Factsheet for Families. Available at: http://costs.adoption.com/articles/the-costs-of-adopting-a-factsheet-for-families.html.

S. L. Cooper and E. S. Glazer. *Choosing Assisted Reproduction: Social Emotional Ethical Considerations.* Perspectives Press, 1998.

T. M. Erickson and M. Lathus. *Assisted Reproduction: The Complete Guide to Having a Baby with the Help of a Third Party.* iUniverse, 2005.

D. D. Gray. *Attaching in Adoption.* Perspectives Press, 2002.

S. Ziegler. *Pathways to Parenthood: The Ultimate Guide to Surrogacy.* BrownWalker Press, 2004.

WE WERE A MARRIED COUPLE with one child and we wanted to have more children. Eight months after our daughter was born, I was diagnosed with premature menopause. I went to a fertility specialist who told me that I had less than a 5 percent chance of becoming pregnant with the fertility treatments she was willing to try. We were at a loss for what to do. It had taken us 15 months to conceive our daughter and we remembered that roller coaster ride all too well. Neither of us wanted to go through the anguish of trying to conceive again when the odds were against us. Instead, we decided to adopt.

We wanted to adopt an infant, so we went to a private agency that was local to us. It took us a whole year to complete the application, and after finishing the paperwork we were devastated to learn that we may be waiting five years to get a call about an available infant. We started to make inquires about international adoption, but then we got a call from the domestic agency. It had only been six months since completing our paperwork. A baby boy had been born, and the agency wanted to know if we were interested in adopting him. We had only a few days to set up the baby room, and a week after our son was born he came home to his family. Seven years have passed and not once have we regretted our decision. Our son is as much a part of our family as if I had given birth to him. He is not our adopted son, he is our son.

Chapter 17

LEGAL CONSIDERATIONS

Most pathways to becoming a parent have some legal issues that need to be considered. Early fertility assistance methods (hormone stimulation and inseminations) are least likely to require legal involvement, provided the sperm used for insemination are from the male partner in the couple wanting to achieve pregnancy. When the more aggressive and invasive assisted reproductive technology (ART) methods are used, complex legal issues can arise. Some forms of ART present more complicated legal issues than others, but each procedure carries its own significant legal considerations. All procedures involve some type of contract that the woman or couple must enter into.

Laws governing the various forms of ART vary greatly from state to state. Depending on the state, the contract signed may not have the intended legal effect, so the people signing the contract must be sure that they understand the full ramifications of the contract before proceeding. It is extremely important to obtain legal advice from an attorney who is competent in assisted reproduction law and thoroughly familiar with the specific state's laws. People seeking legal assistance should interview an attorney carefully to determine his or her experience and familiarity with assisted reproduction law. Because of the great diversity of state laws, this chapter does not attempt to explain the laws of each state. Rather, we focus on the issues you must consider and provide some guidance that will help you to have a meaningful discussion with a qualified attorney.

Generally speaking, the fewer parties involved, the less complicated are the legal issues. Where a couple is able to achieve pregnancy through in vitro fertilization (IVF) using the man's sperm and the woman's eggs, and the woman is able to carry the pregnancy herself, parentage will not be an issue. The couple must still consider what to do with the excess embryos, but there is little risk of custody problems. As the number of participants increases, the complexity of the legal issues increases. With two intended parents, an egg donor, a sperm donor, and a surrogate, the issues of parentage, custody, contracts, and state regulations become particularly complicated. Amazingly, despite the uncertain legal landscape and the vying interests of multiple parties, most assisted reproduction arrangements do go smoothly. Gail Dutton, the author of *A Matter of Trust: The Guide to Gestational Surrogacy*, cites data from the Organization of Parents through Surrogacy: of the more than 8,000 surrogate births recorded in the United States between the mid-1970s and early 1990s, only 17 cases went to court. Proper medical, psychological, and legal counseling prior to embarking on an assisted reproduction procedure can help ensure a positive experience.

All adoptions, too, involve legal issues, which is fairly clear given that a child is being placed in a home to be raised by nonbiological parents. Adoptions can involve a significant amount of legal work, although the complexity varies with the type of adoption.

FERTILITY ASSISTANCE USING YOUR OWN EGGS AND SPERM

The main issue to consider with IVF when a couple uses their own eggs and sperm is what to do with excess embryos created by the procedure. Couples who intend to have more children can have the embryos preserved for their exclusive use in the future. Embryos may also be donated to other infertile couples, or they may be destroyed. These choices raise highly emotional and religious issues for many people. Some people may have strong convictions against destruction, while others are not willing to donate the embryos because doing so would result in their biological child being born to and reared by someone else.

People who choose to donate their embryos have to consider issues of legal parentage for any children resulting from the donated embryos. Some states have statutes relieving donors of parental responsibilities. For example, a Texas statute states clearly that a donor is not the legal parent of a child conceived through assisted reproduction. Despite such statutes, people who choose to donate their embryos will probably be asked to sign a formal relinquishment of parental rights. A formal relinquishment provides extra assurance to all parties that a donor will neither attempt to exercise parental rights nor have parental responsibilities forced upon him or her. A formal relinquishment severs any possible parental ties between the donor and child.

Couples, whether married or not, must also consider what will happen to cryopreserved embryos in the event of divorce or the death of one or both partners. If a couple divorces or splits up, would either spouse have the right to use the stored embryos to have more children? If so, the couple must decide whether the former spouse would have any parental rights or responsibilities toward the children. If not, the couple must decide whether the remaining embryos would be destroyed or donated. Similarly, if one spouse dies, would the remaining spouse be able to use the stored embryos, and if not, would the embryos be destroyed or donated?

While the issue of postdivorce and postdeath use of frozen embryos can be addressed with a contract, there is a risk that the contract wouldn't be fully enforced. Courts have struggled with balancing the rights of each party when couples disagree over the disposition of frozen embryos. While some courts look to contracts for guidance regarding the parties' original intent, other types of legal analysis are often used. Decisions usually turn on whether the court views the embryos as people or as marital property. If the court views the embryos as people, a "best interests of the child" analysis will control the decision. Higher courts have generally overturned these decisions, however. Some courts have treated frozen embryos as marital property, but most courts are reluctant to classify embryos as mere property.

The current trend is to treat embryos as neither people nor property and to use a constitutional analysis in determining the disposition of the embryos. Under the U.S. Constitution, individuals have a right to procreate and a corresponding right not to procreate. In a case where a couple signs an agreement allowing the future use of frozen embryos and one spouse later changes his or her mind and objects to their use, some courts have found that enforcing the prior agreement is against public policy and/or violates a person's constitutional right not to procreate. Despite prior contracts, consent to embryo transfer can usually be revoked by any donor at any time prior to the transfer. Therefore, each transfer requires the consent of all parties.

The issue of using frozen embryos is somewhat clearer in the event of the death of one spouse. Generally, the use of frozen embryos produced from the eggs or sperm of a deceased person is not allowed unless he or she made express instructions before death. The Consent for Cryopreservation contract should address this issue, but it may also be addressed in the person's Last Will and Testament. In a will, a person may bequeath his or her frozen sperm or eggs to a spouse (or to anyone else) for use after the person's death. If the will clearly gives permission and identifies the person who is granted permission, there are no other legal prohibitions on posthumous embryo transfer or IVF. Anyone who has embryos or gametes cryopreserved should have a will drafted that addresses the issue of posthumous use.

In addition to indicating the fate of frozen embryos or gametes, the contracts people must sign with their fertility clinic include information about their rights and responsibilities toward the clinic and the clinic's obligations to them, including storage and disposal of the embryos. They also include provisions for remedies in case of a breach by one party. Like other ART contracts, these contracts are subject to different laws from state to state, so anyone preparing to sign such a contract should first review it carefully with legal counsel.

FERTILITY ASSISTANCE USING DONORS

Donor Sperm

Many states have statutes that deny parental status to sperm and egg donors. In the case of donor sperm, the manner in which a woman pursues insemination can be important. The use of an intermediary, such as a sperm bank, may alter or affect the rights of both the donor and the recipient. For example, a California statute says that if a man gives his sperm to a licensed physician for use in artificial insemination of a woman who is not his wife, then the law treats the man as if he were not the natural (biological) father of the child conceived. But, if he gives the sperm directly to the woman for a self-administered artificial insemination, then the man who donated the sperm is the legal father of the resulting child.

There may be some situations where ART participants want donors to have parental rights, such as when a trusted friend donates sperm to an unmarried woman. The donor may want to have a parental relationship with the child and may insist on it as a condition of providing sperm. In this situation, a co-parenting agreement between the donor and the recipient can allow for such a relationship, even where statutes say that donors are not legal parents.

Donor Eggs

A formal adoption is not generally needed for egg donation. An intended mother giving birth to a child conceived with a donor egg is the presumed mother, so it is unnecessary to amend the birth certificate. However, people who choose to use donor eggs need to have an egg donor contract drafted. To help ensure that the contract is properly executed, the intended parents should make sure that the donor receives independent legal counsel. The contract should address the intended parents' financial obligations surrounding medical care for the donor during the donation process and medical problems the donor may have after the donation (such as ovarian hyperstimulation syndrome). The contract should also include the donor's relinquishment of parental rights. As discussed above, some states have statutes to relieve donors of parental rights, but having the relinquishment specified in the contract provides added assurance to all parties. Lastly, the contract should address what to do with extra embryos.

Donor Embryos

As ART becomes more common, more states are enacting statutes about embryo donation. Embryo "adoption agencies" are also being created to match donors and recipients and to facilitate embryo "adoptions." While these agencies refer to the process as adoption, laws governing traditional child adoptions do not apply to embryo adoptions. At present, there are few statutes specifically addressing embryo donation. Rather, embryo donation is treated in the same way as egg or sperm donation. Where statutes exist, they usually relieve the donor or donors of all parental rights and responsibilities for the children born as a result of their donated gametes or embryos. In some instances, statutes require donors to formally relinquish parental rights. The existence of these statutes implies that embryo donation is legally acceptable. Some states require that extra embryos be preserved for adoption. For example, a Louisiana statute declares that embryos are people under the law and appoints the physician who performed the IVF procedure as temporary guardian of the embryos.

All embryo donors and recipients should seek separate, independent legal representation to draft an agreement addressing the issues surrounding embryo donation. These issues include:

- The donor's relinquishment of parental rights
- The parties' respective rights and obligations toward one another and toward the child
- The possibility of future contact
- The terms of reimbursement

State laws and the specific needs and circumstances of each party should dictate the precise terms of the contract.

USING A SURROGATE

Surrogacy is probably the most legally complex form of assisted reproduction. Three to five parties are usually involved, and an agreement that protects them all must be negotiated and drafted. Part of the complexity of surrogacy arrangements is due to the many different legal aspects that need to be considered, including contract, property, family, and constitutional laws.

Surrogacy is still very controversial, and there is no legal standard for surrogacy from state to state. The Uniform Parentage Act of 2002 was drafted, approved, and recommended by the National Conference of Commissioners on Uniform State Laws. The Act authorizes gestational surrogacy but bans traditional surrogacy. It also sets up a procedure for judicial validation of the agreement, which means that a court must approve the contract before it is enforceable. Although traditional surrogacy agreements are not allowed under the Act, a gestational surrogate may be paid for her services, provided other requirements are met. However, the Uniform Parentage Act serves only as a recommendation. Each state legislature may adopt or reject it, or may enact a revised version.

State legislatures have taken vastly different approaches to surrogacy, with some considering it to be an outright criminal activity and others accepting it virtually unconditionally. Some states have no statutes addressing surrogacy, while others have written statutes that allow surrogacy agreements and place various conditions and restrictions on the practice. Surrogacy also raises constitutional issues of the rights to privacy, to procreate (or not to procreate), and to equal protection. Statutes governing surrogacy may be subject to constitutional challenges, meaning that if a state legislature enacts a statute that violates the U.S. Constitution, a federal court may strike it down.

The two main issues that surrogacy statutes address are (1) the difference between traditional and gestational surrogacy, and (2) whether or not a surrogate can be paid for her services. Most states that have passed surrogacy legislation favor gestational surrogacy. Because a traditional surrogate is also the biological mother of the child, courts have been reluctant to force a traditional surrogate to honor her agreement to relinquish parental rights. Long before surrogacy was possible, adoption law had to grapple with the issue of relinquishment of parental rights to a biological child. In an adoption, the birth mother has a certain amount of time after the child is born to change her mind and keep her child. Because traditional surrogacy, like adoption, requires a birth mother to surrender her biological child, some states have applied adoption laws to allow a traditional surrogate the same opportunity to change her mind. Following from this idea, some surrogacy statutes only recognize surrogacy arrangements where the surrogate is not the biological mother (that is, she is a gestational surrogate).

The second issue is whether or not surrogates should be paid for their services. Every state has a slightly different take on what is acceptable. For example, in Michigan and Washington State, paid surrogacy is a criminal offense. Participants are guilty of a misdemeanor punishable by a fine of up to $10,000 and one year in prison, and facilitators, such as agencies and attorneys, are guilty of a felony punishable by a fine of up to $50,000 and/or imprisonment for up to five years. On the other hand, unpaid surrogacy is not a criminal offense in Michigan, but surrogacy contracts are void and unenforceable. Custody disputes over children born under surrogacy agreements in Michigan are determined under a "best interests of the child" analysis.

Some state statutes impose a blanket prohibition on all surrogacy agreements whether paid or unpaid, while others enforce agreements where the surrogate is unpaid. In Arizona and New York State, all surrogacy contracts are void and unenforceable. By contrast, in Louisiana and Washington State, legislation voids only those surrogacy contracts that provide compensation to the surrogate.

Surrogacy statutes, where they exist, usually place conditions on surrogacy contracts. For example, Texas and Florida both require a medical finding that the intended mother is unable to carry a pregnancy to term. These states also require that the intended parents be married to each other. This requirement precludes unmarried heterosexual couples and homosexual couples from entering surrogacy arrangements as intended parents but does not necessarily exclude would-be single parents. Elsewhere, the Arkansas surrogacy statute recognizes the validity of surrogacy agreements and does not distinguish between traditional and gestational surrogacy. It also allows for single parenting through surrogacy.

For people who want to set up a surrogacy arrangement, the first step is to obtain a well-drafted agreement that complies with their state's laws. The agreement must be in place prior to undergoing either the insemination or the IVF procedure. Under no circumstances should an insemination or an embryo transfer proceed before the legal work has been completed. Because surrogacy is still controversial and state laws vary so greatly, people who do go ahead with a surrogate pregnancy before completing the legal work could thrust themselves into complicated, expensive, and heartbreaking legal problems.

Though it might be subject to certain restrictions, in most states surrogacy is legal. Whether or not surrogacy may be used depends not only on whether a state has surrogacy legislation but also on judicial opinions, precedents, and the facts of the intended parents' particular circumstances. If you think that surrogacy is an avenue you'd like to explore, speak with a lawyer who is well versed in your state's surrogacy laws. A good lawyer will be able to advise you about the best course of action to pursue in your state.

DOMESTIC ADOPTION

Adoptions require a legal proceeding to terminate the birth parents' parental rights and give those rights to the adoptive parents. Therefore, legal representation is always needed for the adoptive family, and separate legal representation for the birth parent or parents is recommended. Unless declared unfit, a birth parent must consent to release the child for adoption. Two states (Alabama and Hawaii) allow the birth mother to consent before the birth, although she must reaffirm her consent after birth. In most states, the birth mother must wait 48 to 72 hours after giving birth before she consents to adoption. In some states the period can be several days to weeks.

Birth fathers with properly established paternity also have the right to consent, and they can generally consent at any time. Several states have laws establishing putative father registries to identify and protect the rights of nonmarital fathers. In states where there is a putative father registry, the birth father must register within a specific time period to preserve his rights.

The period of time during which birth parents can revoke their decision ranges from 3 to 21 days. Some states do not allow birth parents to change their decision, but other states allow revocation under specific circumstances, generally with evidence of fraud, duress, undue influence, coercion, or misrepresentation. The birth parents' consent is irrevocable once the final adoption decree has been issued by the court.

Both the birth mother and the birth father can have their rights to consent terminated if they are found to be unfit parents. If neither birth parent is available, other legal entities, such as the agency that has custody of the child, can have the legal authority to consent. Most states require older children (those over ten to fourteen years old, depending on the state) to consent to their adoption, if they are mentally able to do so.

Agency adoptions are legal in all 50 states. Independent or nonagency adoptions are legal in all but four states (Colorado, Delaware, Massachusetts, and Connecticut). Some states do not allow people who are unlicensed to advertise for independent adoptions, so only licensed adoption agencies can advertise. These states include California, Delaware, Georgia, Hawaii, Idaho, Illinois, Kansas, Kentucky, Massachusetts, Montana, Nebraska, Nevada, North Carolina, North Dakota, Ohio, Rhode Island, and Wisconsin. However, residents of these states may still advertise in out-of-state publications that are read in their state and in national publications such as *USA Today*.

The recent trend of allowing open adoptions, in which a child can contact his or her birth parents, is gaining more and more acceptance. A recent review done by the Evan B. Donaldson Adoption Institute recommends that all states establish legally enforceable postadoption contact agreements, but to date, only 13 states have established such policies. People who are considering a domestic adoption need to consider their state's policy on open adoption and whether or not they would be willing to allow contact between their adopted child and the child's birth parents.

Adoption policies and procedures are governed at the state level and may vary from state to state. Generally, however, a home study by a licensed social worker must be completed prior to the final adoption proceeding. The social worker will interview the prospective parents, visit and inspect the home, conduct background checks (including criminal background and financial and credit checks), and make a recommendation to the court as to whether or not the prospective parents are suitable. After the home study is complete and any required waiting periods have expired, a final adoption hearing is held in which the court approves the adoption and signs the final decree. A hearing to terminate the parental rights of the birth parents may be held before, or at the same time as, the final adoption hearing.

INTERNATIONAL ADOPTION

Every country has its own set of legal restrictions on who may and may not adopt a child. In particular, gay and lesbian couples and single applicants can have difficulty adopting internationally. The services of an adoption agency are key to navigating the legal issues in the country of interest.

The Child Citizenship Act of 2001 streamlined INS procedures for acquiring U.S. citizenship for internationally adopted children. A child who has been fully and finally adopted in his or her birth country by an American citizen will be admitted to the United States as an immigrant and will automatically acquire U.S. citizenship. As described in chapter 15, the INS issues a certificate of citizenship after appropriate forms are filed. A qualified immigration attorney should be consulted to ensure that a child's citizenship is properly obtained.

Although a child adopted abroad and escorted to the United States by the adoptive parent does not need to be readopted, many people do readopt in the United States. U.S. adoption documents are easier to read in American schools and courts, and attorneys may recommend readoption to protect inheritance rights. Readoption laws are governed by the individual states.

LEGAL ISSUES FOR GAYS AND LESBIANS

Of all couples who decide to have children, gay and lesbian relationships are the most complicated from a legal standpoint. Gay and lesbian parenting is extremely controversial. Parenting contracts that would be upheld if the intended parents were heterosexual may not be if the intended parents are gay or lesbian. To date, there are very few statutes or court opinions that deal specifically with gay and lesbian adoptions.

Gay and lesbian couples have a host of issues to consider before attempting to build a family through assisted reproduction. Parenting agreements can address issues of parental rights, financial responsibility, guardianship in the event of the death of a partner, and custody in the event of the relationship ending. However, these agreements may or may not be upheld in court. Because gays and lesbians who want to be parents face such difficult legal issues, it is imperative that they seek the advice of a competent attorney in the very early stages of the process. An attorney can help not only in documenting and executing the assisted reproduction plan, but in creating a parenting plan that works and is within legal boundaries.

A woman may achieve pregnancy through artificial insemination using donor sperm, but her lesbian partner will likely have no parental rights. A woman who gives birth is the presumed mother and is named on the child's birth certificate as the mother. While husbands have paternity rights, a nonbiological mother in a lesbian relationship usually does not have parental rights. Even where one partner donates the eggs and the other carries the pregnancy, one partner may find she has no parental rights. The part-

ner who donated the eggs may file a lawsuit to prove her maternity, but such a lawsuit creates a risk that the nonbiological
mother (the one who carried the pregnancy) may be viewed only
as a surrogate and won't have any parental rights. Some states allow the nonbiological mother to become a legal parent through a
stepparent adoption or give the nonbiological mother rights as a
de facto parent. However, some states, such as Florida, expressly
prohibit such adoptions.

Gay men may father a child with the help of a surrogate and
donor eggs or embryos. These types of arrangements require a surrogacy agreement. While a surrogacy agreement can name both
partners as the intended parents, many state laws prohibit such
arrangements. Generally, the legal father will be the partner who
contributed the sperm and the other partner will have no parental
rights.

With respect to adoption, state laws run the gamut from expressly allowing gays and lesbians to adopt to expressly prohibit-
ing their doing so. In 2000, 49 states allowed adoptions by gays
and lesbians, but this number has since decreased. Currently, gays
and lesbians are allowed to adopt in every state except Florida,
Mississippi, and Utah. However, additional states are considering laws to make adoption by gays and lesbians illegal. International adoptions are nearly impossible for gay and lesbian couples.
Some countries even require prospective parents to write a formal statement declaring that they are heterosexual.

FURTHER READING

Adoption.com. Statutes at a Glance: Consent to Adoption—Laws. Available at:
    http://laws.adoption.com.
adoption.org. National Adoption Clearinghouse. Available at: www.adoption
    .org/adopt/national-adoption-clearinghouse.php.
L. Beauvais-Godwin and R. Godwin. *The Complete Adoption: Everything You
    Need to Know to Adopt a Child.* Adams Media, 2000.
G. Dutton. *A Matter of Trust: The Guide to Gestational Surrogacy.* Clouds Pub-
    lishing, 1997.

J. N. Erichsen and H. R. Erichsen. *How to Adopt Internationally: A Guide for Agency-Directed and Independent Adoptions.* Mesa House, 2003.

T. M. Erickson and M. Lathus. *Assisted Reproduction: The Complete Guide to Having a Baby with the Help of a Third Party.* iUniverse, 2005.

E. S. Glazer and E. W. Sterling. *Having Your Baby through Egg Donation.* Perspectives Press, 2003.

Human Rights Campaign. Surrogacy Laws: State by State. 2004. Available at: http://www.hrc.org.

R. Mintzer. *Yes, You Can Adopt! A Comprehensive Guide to Adoption.* Avalon, Carroll and Graf, 2003.

G. Sutton. *A Matter of Trust: The Guide to Gestational Surrogacy.* Clouds Publishing, 1997.

O. R. Sweet and P. Bryan. *Adopt International: Everything You Need to Know to Adopt a Child from Abroad.* Noonday Press, 1996.

TASC: The American Surrogacy Center. www.surrogacy.com.

C. F. Vercollone, H. Moss, and R. Moss. *Helping the Stork.* Macmillan, 1997.

I'VE ALWAYS KNOWN that I wanted to be a father, and because I'm a gay man, I always imagined that I would adopt a child. Two years ago I did become a father, but instead of being adopted, my daughter was born with the help of an egg donor and a surrogate. The two women who helped my partner and me become parents are close friends of ours. They are a lesbian couple, and each has a child from a previous relationship.

My partner and I first started talking seriously about having a child about five years ago. We looked into all the possibilities for adoption but were daunted by a few aspects. For a domestic adoption, we were concerned about birth mothers not taking us seriously as possible parents for their child. We thought it might be difficult to portray a male couple with no child-rearing experience as nurturing parents. We knew we'd have to compete, as it were, with other couples wanting to adopt. For an international adoption, we were aware that several countries would not accept us as adoptive parents. Most of all, though, we were concerned about placing too much on a child of another nationality (especially when the child became a teen). We're both Caucasian, and we think that any child we raise will have enough to think about by having two fathers, let alone grappling with having two fathers of a different race.

In the midst of our discussions about whether we would go ahead with applying to an adoption agency, my partner suddenly suggested that perhaps we should think about using a surrogate. This possibility had never occurred to me. When our friends offered to help us, whereby one would provide an egg and the other would carry the pregnancy, the possibility of having a child by surrogacy began to seem feasible. We decided that we would go ahead and that I would provide the sperm, because I'm quite a bit younger than my partner.

We all agreed (and had legal documents drawn up) that my partner and I would be the parents and principal caregivers of the child, and that our friends, the egg donor and the surrogate, would be as involved in the child's life as close friends or aunts might be. My partner and I were very much a part of our surrogate's pregnancy; we saw her and her partner every week and went to some of the medical appointments. Going to an ultrasound appointment was the moment that really brought home to me that we were going to have a child. When our daughter was born, we got her onto a bottle immediately and the surrogate expressed breast milk for us to feed her with. This arrangement went on for six months, then we weaned her to formula.

We're incredibly grateful to our friends for giving us the opportunity to be parents, and we're so happy to have them remain a part of our and our daughter's life. We intend to tell our daughter right from a young age how she was conceived. We don't want her biological mother and pregnancy mother to be strangers to her.

Chapter 18

FINAL THOUGHTS

We hope that the information and personal stories in this book have given you a better idea of what to expect with each option for becoming a parent. Ideally, you would have been able to identify which pathways are realistic for you. So, where do you go from here? Two key factors that are likely to influence how you proceed are time and money. Although you probably want a child immediately, it is helpful to plan a range of time that is acceptable to you and your partner or spouse and then determine the amount of money you can afford to spend during that time.

When you've decided how much time and money you are willing or able to spend, you can determine your strategy. First, identify the pathway or pathways that you want to pursue, and then decide what your stopping points will be for each pathway. If a particular pathway is not bringing success for you, having a clear stopping point will help you avoid emotional and financial exhaustion. Figure out exactly how far you want to go, or can afford to go, before you abandon the pathway and switch to another, or decide to stop altogether. For example, how many in vitro fertilization attempts or birth mother contacts will you make before moving on to another choice with a higher chance for success, such as donor eggs or international adoption? Will you stop after trying a certain pathway and live child-free, or will you move on to a different pathway? The best approach is to be prepared with a backup plan so that you have another option to pursue if a particular pathway doesn't work out.

Once you have decided on your strategy, obtain as much information as you can about the pathway or pathways in your plan from the internet, books, and other resources. Now is the time to get the "how to" information. Then, armed with information, you are ready to set your plan in motion. As you do, try to remember that nearly everyone can become a parent, one way or another, and no matter how exhausting the process may seem, parents universally agree that it is worth it.

ACKNOWLEDGMENTS

The authors are deeply thankful to the following individuals for their contributions to the book: Lynne Bonner, Stephanie Broyles, Jennifer Ericson, Jane Hitti, Patty Kissinger, Toni Newton, Paulette Penn, Carol Pindaro, Bob and Maggie Post, and Rowena Rae.

Appendixes

APPENDIX A

Summary of Your Influence on Genetic Background and Fetal and Infant Environments

Pathway	Degree of influence	Genetic background	Age of child
Fertility assistance			
Own eggs and sperm	High	Yes	Conception
Donor eggs or sperm	High	Yes	Conception
Donor embryos	Moderate	No	Embryo
Traditional surrogacy	Moderate	Yes	Newborn
Gestational surrogacy	Moderate	Yes	Newborn
Adoption			
Domestic agency	Low	No	Newborn, young children
Domestic independent	Moderate	No	Newborn
International	Low	No	Infants, young children

APPENDIX B

Environmental Influence, by Child's Age and Type of Adoption

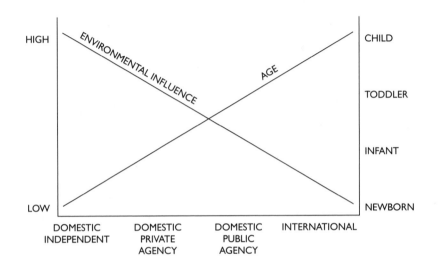

APPENDIX C

Summary of Pregnancy and Medical Risks

Pathway	Risks
Fertility assistance	
Own eggs and sperm	Fertility intervention risks including ovarian hyperstimulation; pregnancy risks; risks associated with multiple birth
	Chromosomal abnormalities more frequent among couples using intracytoplasmic sperm injection
	Possibly a slightly increased risk for congenital malformations with assisted reproductive technology (controversial)
Donor sperm	Pregnancy risks
Donor eggs	Pregnancy risks; risks associated with multiple birth
Donor embryos	Pregnancy risks; risks associated with multiple birth
Traditional surrogacy	—
Gestational surrogacy	Fertility intervention risks for the intended mother and possible risks associated with multiple birth for the carrier
Adoption	
Domestic public agency	Fetal drug/alcohol exposure
Domestic private agency	Possible fetal drug/alcohol exposure
Domestic independent	—
International	Fetal drug/alcohol exposure; attention-deficit/hyperactivity disorder; malnutrition; growth developmental problems; lack of medical records; anemia; selected infectious diseases

Note: A dash (—) indicates that, on a population basis, there is probably no increased risk compared with the general population.

APPENDIX D

Summary of Mental Health Risks

Pathway	*Risks*
Fertility assistance	
Own eggs and sperm	Risks associated with multiple birth, including prematurity and developmental delays
Donor sperm	—
Donor eggs	Risks associated with multiple birth, as above
Donor embryos	Risks associated with multiple birth, as above
Traditional surrogacy	—
Gestational surrogacy	Risks associated with multiple birth, as above
Adoption choices	
Domestic public agency	Fetal drug/alcohol exposure; attachment disorders; attention-deficit/hyperactivity disorder (ADHD)
Domestic private agency	Possible fetal drug/alcohol exposure; possible attachment disorders; possible ADHD—all depending on characteristics of biological mother and age of infant at adoption
Domestic independent	—
International	Fetal drug/alcohol exposure; attachment disorders; ADHD; malnutrition; growth developmental problems

Note: A dash (—) indicates that, on a population basis, there is probably no increased risk compared with the general population.

APPENDIX E

Summary of Emotional Risks

Pathway	Risks
Fertility assistance	
Own eggs and sperm	Effect of hormones; effect on sex life; contraceptive failures; miscarriage
Donor sperm	Contraceptive failures; miscarriage; no paternal genetic connection; possible long-term concerns regarding questions about biological father
Donor eggs	Contraceptive failures; miscarriage; no maternal genetic connection; possible long-term concerns regarding questions about biological mother
Donor embryos	Contraceptive failures; miscarriage; no maternal or paternal genetic connection; possible long-term concerns regarding questions about biological parents
Traditional surrogacy	Contraceptive failures; miscarriage; no maternal genetic connection; surrogate may not relinquish parental rights; unable to experience pregnancy
Gestational surrogacy	Effect of hormones; contraceptive failures; miscarriage; unable to experience pregnancy
Adoption	
Domestic public agency	Unable to experience pregnancy; may need to make decision about adoption of special needs child in short time period
Domestic private agency	Unable to experience pregnancy; may need to "sell self" to potential birth mother; need to maintain good relationship with birth mother; adoption disruption
Domestic independent	Unable to experience pregnancy; need to find birth mother; may need to "sell self" to potential birth mother; need to maintain good relationship with birth mother; adoption disruption

(continued)

Pathway	Risks
International	Unable to experience pregnancy; adoption disruption; may need to make decision about adoption of special needs child quickly, without American expert opinion

APPENDIX F

Summary of Time from Start of Process to Conception (Fertility Assistance) or Becoming a Parent (Adoption)

Pathway	Time
Fertility assistance	
Own eggs, using ART[1]	6 months to 2 years
Donor sperm[2]	3 months to 1 year
Donor eggs[1]	6 months to 3 years
Donor embryos[1]	1 to 3 years
Surrogacy[1]	1 to 3 years
Adoption	
Domestic public agency[3]	6 months to 9 years
Domestic private agency	9 months to 2 years
Domestic independent[4]	3 months to 5+ years
International	1 to 2 years

1. Does not include time individuals/couples have spent in trying other fertility assistance options.
2. Assumes no maternal fertility problems, including advanced maternal age.
3. Depends on factors such as child ethnicity, special needs status, and so forth.
4. Depends on resources for advertising.

APPENDIX G

Summary of Hassles

Pathway	Hassles
Fertility assistance	Potential travel; no or little flexibility for timing evaluations during active cycles
Surrogacy	Finding a surrogate; attorney and court visits
Adoption	Home study; obtaining multiple notarized documents; preplacement and postplacement interviews; compiling a portfolio and finding a birth mother (independent adoption); travel (international adoption)

APPENDIX H

Summary of Financial Costs

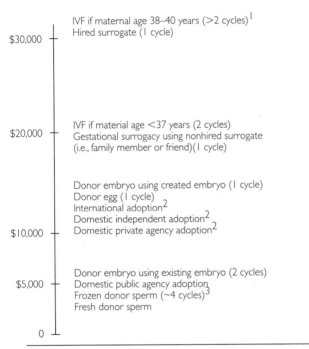

$30,000 — IVF if maternal age 38–40 years (>2 cycles)[1]
Hired surrogate (1 cycle)

$20,000 — IVF if material age <37 years (2 cycles)
Gestational surrogacy using nonhired surrogate
(i.e., family member or friend)(1 cycle)

Donor embryo using created embryo (1 cycle)
Donor egg (1 cycle)
International adoption[2]
Domestic independent adoption[2]
$10,000 — Domestic private agency adoption[2]

Donor embryo using existing embryo (2 cycles)
$5,000 — Domestic public agency adoption
Frozen donor sperm (~4 cycles)[3]
Fresh donor sperm

0

Note: This chart compares average pathway costs for choices having a 50 percent or higher chance of success.

1. If maternal age is over 40 years, multiple cycles are needed and costs will exceed $70,000.

2. With the exception of public agencies, adoption costs can be highly variable. Shown here are the lower estimates.

3. Assumes a maternal age less than 35 years.

APPENDIX I

Summary of Legal Considerations

Pathway	Legal considerations
Fertility assistance	
Own eggs and sperm	Embryo disposition; contract with fertility clinic
Donor sperm	Manner in which insemination is done; relinquishment of donor's parental rights
Donor eggs	Contract with donor; relinquishment of donor's parental rights; embryo disposition
Donor embryos	Contract with donors; relinquishment of donor's parental rights
Surrogacy	Contract with surrogate; relinquishment of surrogate's parental rights; judicial validation of surrogacy contract; amending birth certificate; state laws regarding restrictions and conditions on surrogacy arrangements
Adoption	
Domestic agency	Consent from birth mother (or birth parents) and possibly from child; finalizing adoption
Domestic independent	Need to know state laws; finding birth mother; consent from birth mother (or birth parents); finalizing adoption
International	Need to know country laws; readoption in United States

GLOSSARY

abruptio placentae: A condition in which the placenta separates early from the uterus and causes bleeding that can result in fetal complications or death.

adoption agency: A business incorporated as a nonprofit or for-profit entity and licensed by the state to place children for adoption and/or to conduct home studies.

adoption disruption: Termination of an adoption process after the child is placed in an adoptive home and before the adoption is legally finalized. The child returns to the birth parent(s), goes into foster care, or is placed with new adoptive parents.

adoption dissolution: Termination of an adoption after it is legally finalized, usually because the birth mother changes her mind after the adoption and goes through the court to obtain her biological child.

agency-facilitated adoption: An adoption in which the agency introduces adoptive parents to a birth mother before the baby's birth. Unless the agency receives outside funds, the adoptive parents pay the birth mother's legal, living, and counseling expenses (as in nonagency adoptions) in addition to the agency fee.

alcohol-related neurodevelopmental disorder (ARND): A condition in which a child is easily stressed and can have difficulty establishing sleeping patterns, toilet training, and personal space.

Americans with Disabilities Act (ADA): A federal civil rights act that protects individuals with disabilities, including people with HIV/AIDS or hepatitis. One ADA provision is that adoption agencies may not use "standards or criteria or methods of discrimination that have the effect of discriminating on the basis of disability."

amniocentesis: A test in which amniotic fluid (the fluid around the fetus) is aspirated at 15 to 18 weeks gestation to check the fetus for genetic abnormalities.

assisted reproductive technology (ART): A fertility treatment in which both the eggs and sperm are handled in a laboratory. The most common ART method is in vitro fertilization (IVF).

attachment disorder: A mental health disorder with the following symptoms: self-destructive behavior, learning problems, fire setting, and cruelty to siblings, animals, and others. People with an attachment disorder may lie, have an underdeveloped conscience, and be fascinated with weapons, blood, or gore.

attention deficit disorder (ADD): A mental health disorder in which a person's brain does not sustain attention on the main point of an activity or a conversation. The brain seems to get "stuck" on a particular topic or particular behavioral pattern. People with ADD have a hard time maintaining self-control or thinking ahead.

attention-deficit/hyperactivity disorder (ADHD): A mental health disorder in which ADD (see above) is combined with hyperactivity.

azoospermia: A condition in which a man produces no sperm.

blastocyst: An embryo that is about five days old and consists of around 60 to 100 cells.

cervix: The opening of the uterus.

Children of Lesbians and Gays Everywhere (COLAGE): One of several national support groups geared to the estimated 250,000 children of gay couples and the millions of other children in the United States with a gay parent.

chorionic villus sampling (CVS): A test in which the placenta is biopsied to check for genetic abnormalities in the fetus. CVS is an alternative to amniocentesis and can be done earlier in the pregnancy (at 10 to 13 weeks).

Clomid: A medication that stimulates egg production. Clomid is a brand name (Serophene is another); clomiphene citrate is the generic name.

Clomid challenge test: A test to determine if a woman has adequate "ovarian reserve" (a sufficient number of good-quality eggs). A Clomid challenge test is most frequently done for women over thirty-five years of age.

closed adoption: An adoption in which the birth parents and adoptive parents never meet. The adoptive parents complete all the necessary steps for adoption, and then the agency calls them to take home a baby who has been released for adoption.

conception: The fertilization of an egg by a sperm to create an embryo.

controlled ovarian hyperstimulation: Injection of a woman with hormones called gonadotropins to increase the number of egg follicles that develop in the ovaries so that more mature eggs are released. The goal is to make more than the one or two mature follicles and eggs that are formed in a natural cycle.

cryopreservation: A process in which cells or tissue are preserved by cooling to subzero temperatures. At these low temperatures all biological activity is stopped. If vitrification techniques are used for cryopreservation, then cell damage due to ice crystal formation is avoided.

cytoplasmic transfer: An ART procedure in which a small amount of cytoplasm (the viscous semifluid inside an egg) is taken from a donor egg and injected into a woman's own egg. The rationale is that the transferred cytoplasm may enhance the quality of a subsequent embryo.

directed donor: A sperm, egg, or embryo donor who is known to the recipients. Also called a known donor.

ectopic pregnancy: Implantation of an embryo in one of the fallopian tubes instead of the uterus. The embryo cannot survive, and sometimes the fallopian tube is damaged or destroyed.

embryo: An egg that has been fertilized by a sperm.

endometriosis: A disorder in which endometrial tissue (which normally lines the uterus and is shed during the menstrual period) is located in various places in the pelvic area outside the uterus. Endometriosis can cause infertility.

estrogen: A hormone involved in egg maturation. Changes in a woman's estrogen level are monitored during fertility treatment to track egg maturation.

fetal alcohol effects (FAE): A condition in which a child has been adversely affected by prenatal alcohol exposure but does not meet the criteria for FAS (see below). Children with FAE may have one or more congenital, central nervous system, behavioral, or cognitive defects or deficits.

fetal alcohol syndrome (FAS): A condition resulting from a baby's exposure to alcohol during the pregnancy. Children with FAS can have slower growth, a smaller head, heart problems, facial abnormalities, central nervous system neurodevelopmental abnormalities (including mental retardation), and a pattern of cognitive and behavioral abnormalities not explained by other factors.

fibroids: Benign tumors arising from the muscle wall of the uterus. They usually do not require treatment, but if they do cause problems, surgical treatment is generally recommended.

follicle: Another name for an immature egg.

follicle-stimulating hormone (FSH): A hormone that stimulates egg production. Women who are going through menopause have high levels of FSH, so FSH levels can be tested to check menopausal status.

gestational surrogate: A woman who carries a pregnancy with eggs donated from the intended mother or an egg donor and sperm donated from the intended father or a sperm donor. The intended parents take custody of the child immediately after delivery. Also called a gestational carrier.

gonadotropins: Hormones given during fertility treatment to stimulate egg production.

home study: An evaluation of an individual's or couple's capability to raise an adopted child. A home study is completed by an adoption agency employee or a social worker.

hyperstimulation syndrome: *See* ovarian hyperstimulation syndrome.

hypospadias: A condition in males in which the opening of the urethra (where the urine leaves the body) is on the underside of the penis.

hysterosalpingogram (HSG): An X-ray test in which dye is injected into the uterus and fallopian tubes. A radiologist can then determine if the tubes are blocked or if there is another cause that may be keeping a woman from getting pregnant.

identified agency adoption: An adoption in which the prospective parents and birth mother have already made an agreement with one another before involving an agency. An identified adoption proceeds like an independent adoption, but the agency provides guidance and the laws governing an agency adoption are followed, rather than those governing an independent adoption. Also called a designated agency adoption.

independent adoption: An adoption in which an agency is not used. Independent adoption entails hiring an attorney who will either locate a birth mother or instruct the prospective parents on how to find one themselves through advertising or networking. Also called nonagency, private, or self-directed adoption.

intracervical insemination (ICI): A procedure in which sperm are inserted just inside the cervical opening. ICI is so simple that it can be done at home.

intracytoplasmic sperm injection (ICSI): An assisted reproductive technology procedure in which a single sperm is injected into an egg.

intrauterine insemination (IUI): A procedure in which sperm are inserted through the cervix and into the uterus, using a thin, flexible catheter. The sperm must be washed prior to IUI.

in vitro fertilization (IVF): An assisted reproductive technology procedure in which eggs are fertilized by sperm in a dish in a laboratory.

laparoscopy: A surgical procedure that involves inserting a lighted telescope and other instruments into the abdomen through a very small incision. The procedure requires anesthesia but can be done in an outpatient clinic. Laparoscopy is often used to diagnose and treat endometriosis.

luteinizing hormone (LH): A hormone involved in egg maturation. LH levels are monitored during fertility treatments to track how the eggs are maturing.

microcephaly: A condition in a newborn characterized by a smaller than normal head.

multiple gestation: A pregnancy with more than one fetus in the uterus.

nonagency adoption: *See* independent adoption.

oligozoospermia: A condition in which a man has a low sperm count.

open adoption: An adoption in which the adoptive parents and the birth mother or birth parents maintain an open line of communication after the adoption has been finalized.

orphan petition: INS form I-600, titled Petition to Classify Orphan as an Immediate Relative. When submitted, form I-600 must be accompanied by several documents to verify a child's status as an orphan.

ovarian hyperstimulation syndrome (OHSS): A condition in which a woman's body overrresponds to hormone stimulation during fertility treatment and her estrogen rises to very high levels. This complication can be dangerous and potentially fatal.

ovulation: The time when an egg (or eggs) is released from the ovary.

percutaneous epididymal sperm aspiration (PESA): A procedure to extract sperm from the epididymis, used in men with a vasectomy or a condition resulting in the absence of sperm in the ejaculate.

placenta previa: A condition in which the placenta is completely or partially covering the opening of the uterus. Placenta previa can cause bleeding during the second or third trimesters, and usually the baby must be delivered by Cesarian section.

polygenic defects: A faulty interaction of two or more genes in the chromosome resulting in the abnormal development of an organ.

postcoital test: A test to determine how well the sperm function in the vaginal environment. A couple is asked to have intercourse around the time of ovulation, and approximately 4 to 12 hours later a sample of mucus is taken from the cervix and examined under a microscope.

pregestational diagnosis (PGD): An assisted reproductive technology procedure in which an embryo biopsy is done, usually on day 3 of laboratory culture when the embryos consist of four to nine cells. The outer layer (zona pellucida) is opened by mechanical, chemical, or laser techniques and one or two cells are removed to test for the most common chromosomal problems. The test results can assist in determining which embryos should be transferred to the uterus.

progesterone: A hormone that is essential for maintaining a pregnancy. Progesterone is given to pregnant women who have conceived with the help of fertility assistance.

public adoption agencies: Adoption agencies that are usually part of the state social services department and primarily place children who have been in the foster care system. The children may or may not have physical health problems. Their biological parents' rights have usually been involuntarily terminated (or are in the process of being terminated) because of abuse or neglect.

putative father registry: A registry that allows the nonmarital biological father of a child to record his interest in the child. The father must be notified of legal proceedings that bear on the well-being of his child.

reactive attachment disorder (RAD): A disorder in which infants and young children have serious problems forming emotional attachments and socially relating with caregivers, peers, and family.

selective reduction: Terminating one or more of several fetuses, either because of a chromosomal, structural, or genetic abnormality or to reduce the number of fetuses in a multiple pregnancy. Also called pregnancy reduction or selective termination.

singleton gestation: A pregnancy in which a woman carries only one fetus.

Society for Assisted Reproductive Technology (SART): An organization affiliated with the American Society for Reproductive Medicine (ASRM). SART's membership consists of approximately four hundred assisted reproductive technology clinics in the United States. SART publishes statistics gathered from its members every year.

special needs: A general term to describe children with characteristics that make their placement in adoptive families more difficult than for other children. Examples of special needs children are older children, children of certain ethnic backgrounds, sibling groups, and children with a disability, medical condition, or psychiatric problem.

sperm washing: A laboratory technique to remove substances called prostaglandins from sperm in preparation for intrauterine insemination.

teratospermia: A descriptive term for sperm samples with a reduced number of normal-appearing sperm.

testicular sperm extraction (TESE): A procedure to extract sperm directly from the testes, used in men with a vasectomy or a condition that results in the absence of sperm in the ejaculate.

traditional adoption: A closed adoption in which the birth and adoptive parents never meet.

traditional surrogacy: A surrogate pregnancy in which the surrogate is both the biological mother and the pregnancy carrier. Either the intended father provides the sperm or donor sperm are used to artificially inseminate the surrogate.

transvaginal ultrasound: An ultrasound done by inserting a long probe into the vagina to evaluate egg development.

vitrification: An ultrarapid cooling technique, different from conventional cryopreservation (freezing), that can be used to preserve eggs and embryos.

X-linked disorder: A type of disorder that occurs only in men who inherit a faulty gene from their mother.

SELECTED REFERENCES

General

Centers for Disease Control and Prevention. 2003 Assisted Reproductive Technology (ART) Report (www.cdc.gov/ART/ART2003).

Centers for Disease Control and Prevention. 2004 Assisted Reproductive Technology (ART) Report (www.cdc.gov/ART/ART2004).

The Evan B. Donaldson Adoption Institute. 1997 Benchmark Adoption Survey: First Public Opinion Survey on American Attitudes toward Adoption (www.adoptioninstitute.org/survey/baexec.html).

Rebar RW, DeCherney AH. Assisted reproductive technology in the United States. *N Engl J Med* 2004;350:1603–4.

Use of assisted reproductive technology—United States, 1996–1998. *MMWR Morb Mortal Wkly Rep* 2002;51:97–101.

Chapter 3. Assisted Reproductive Technology (ART) Using Your Own Eggs or Sperm

Boldt J, Cline D, McLaughlin D. Human oocyte cryopreservation as an adjunct to IVF—embryo transfer cycles. *Hum Reprod* 2003;18:1250–55.

Centers for Disease Control and Prevention. 2003 Assisted Reproductive Technology (ART) Report (data from Society for Assisted Reproductive Technology) (www.cdc.gov/ART/ART2003).

Centers for Disease Control and Prevention. 2004 Assisted Reproductive Technology (ART) Report (www.cdc.gov/ART/ART2004).

Ethics Committee of the American Society for Reproductive Medicine. Sex selection and preimplantation genetic diagnosis. *Fertil Steril* 1999;72:595–98.

Newroth F, Rahimi G, Isachenko E, et al. Cryopreservation in assisted reproductive technology: new trends. *Semin Reprod Med* 2005;23:325–32.

Revel A, Safran A, Laufer N, et al. Twin pregnancy following 12 years of human embryo cryopreservation: case report. *Hum Reprod* 2004;19:328–29.

Yoon TK, Kim TJ, Park SE, et al. Live birth after vitrification in a stimulated in vitro fertilization—embryo transfer program. *Fertil Steril* 2003;79:1323–26.

Chapter 5. Using Donor Eggs and Embryos

Centers for Disease Control and Prevention. 2003 Assisted Reproductive Technology (ART) Report: National Summary (data from Society for Assisted Reproductive Technology) (http://apps.nccd.cdc.gov/ART2003/nation03.asp).

Centers for Disease Control and Prevention. 2004 Assisted Reproductive Technology (ART) Report (www.cdc.gov/ART/ART2004).

Keefe DL, Parry JP. New approaches to assisted reproductive technologies. *Semin Reprod Med* 2005;23:301–9.

Chapter 7. Domestic and International Adoptions

The Evan B. Donaldson Adoption Institute. Foster Care Facts (www.adoption institute.org/FactOverview/foster.html).

Chapter 8. Which Options Are Available to You?

Centers for Disease Control and Prevention. 2003 Assisted Reproductive Technology (ART) Report: National Summary (data from Society for Assisted Reproductive Technology) (http://apps.nccd.cdc.gov/ART2003/nation03.asp).

Centers for Disease Control and Prevention. 2004 Assisted Reproductive Technology (ART) Report: National Summary (data from Society for Assisted Reproductive Technology) (http://apps.nccd.cdc.gov/ART2004/nation04.asp).

Ethics Committee of the American Society for Reproductive Medicine. Child-rearing ability and the provision of fertility services. *Fertil Steril* 2004;82:564–67.

Ethics Committee of the American Society for Reproductive Medicine. Fertility treatment when the prognosis is very poor or futile. *Fertil Steril* 2004;82:806–10.

Practice Committee of the American Society for Reproductive Medicine. Guidelines for the provision of infertility services. *Fertil Steril* 2004; 82:S24–S25.

Chapter 9. Considerations for Nontraditional Families

Americans with Disabilities Act of 1990. S. 933. One Hundred and First Congress of the United States of America at the Second Session, begun and held at the city of Washington on Tuesday, the twenty-third day of January, 1990.

Annas G. Protecting patients from discrimination—the Americans with Disabilities Act and HIV infection. *N Engl J Med* 1998;339:1255–59.

Bragon v Abbott (1998); 524 U.S. 624, 118 S. Ct. 2196.

CWLA: Child Welfare League of America. Americans with Disabilities Act: What Adoption Agencies Need to Know (www.cwla.org/programs/adoption/Americans_with_disabilities.htm).

Ethics Committee of the American Society for Reproductive Medicine. Human immunodeficiency virus. *Fertil Steril* 2002;77:218–22.

Mandelbrot L, Heard I, Henrion-Geant E, Henrion R. Natural conception in HIV-negative women with HIV-infected partners. *Lancet* 1997;349:850–51.

Marina S, Marina F, Alcolea R, et al. HIV type 1-serodiscordant couples can bear healthy children after undergoing intrauterine insemination. *Fertil Steril* 1998;70:35–39.

Peterson L. Court Rules Agencies May Deny Placement Based on Prospective Parent's Disability. CWLA: Child Welfare League of America (www.cwla .org/programs/adoption/Americans_with_disabilities2.htm).

Practice Committee of the American Society for Reproductive Medicine. Hepatitis and reproduction. *Fertil Steril* 2004;82:1754–64.

Semprini AE, Levi-Setti P, Ravizza M, Pari G. Assisted conception to reduce the risk of male-to-female sexual transfer of HIV in serodiscordant couples: an update (abstract). In *Abstracts of the Scientific Oral and Poster Sessions of the 57th Annual Meeting of the ASRM, Orlando, FL, October 20–25, 2001*, S-49.

U.S. Department of Justice. Questions and Answers: The Americans with Disabilities Act and Persons with HIV/AIDS (www.ada.gov/pubs/hivquanda .txt).

Chapter 10. Your Influence on Genetics and the Fetal and Infant Environments

Barth RP, Freundlich M, Brodzinsky D. Alcohol related birth defects and international adoption. In *Adoption and Prenatal Alcohol and Drug Exposure: Research, Policy, and Practice*, ed. RP Barth, M Freundlich, and D Brodzinsky. Arlington, VA: Child Welfare League of America and Evan B. Donaldson Adoption Institute, 2000 (available at: www.orphandoctor.com/services/ preadoptconsult/alcoholrbd.html).

Collins JA. Preimplantation genetic screening in older mothers. *N Engl J Med* 2007;357:61–63.

Hardy K, Wright C, Rice S, et al. Future developments in assisted reproduction in humans. *Reproduction* 2002;123:171–83.

Kearns WG, Pen R, Graham J, et al. Preimplantation genetic diagnosis and screening. *Semin Reprod Med* 2005;23:336–47.

Sermon KD, Michiels A, Harton G, et al. ESHRE PGD Consortium data collection VI: cycles from January to December 2003 with pregnancy follow-up to October 2004. *Hum Reprod* 2007;22:323–36.

Stein MT, Faber S, Berger SP, et al. International adoption: a four-year-old child with unusual behaviors adopted at six months of age. *J Dev Behav Pediatr* 2003;24:63–69.

Chapter 11. Pregnancy and Medical Risks for Mother and Child

adoption.com. Adoption Statistics: Drug Exposure (http://statistics.adoption
.com/drug_exposed_infants.php).

Allen VM, Wilson RD, Cheung A. Pregnancy outcomes after assisted reproductive technology. *J Obstet Gynecol Can* 2006;28:220–50.

Beidso JM, Johnston BD. Preparing families for international adoption. *Pediatr
Rev* 2004;25:242–49.

Boone JL, Hostetter MK, Weitzman CC. The predictive accuracy of preadoption video review in adoptees from Russian and Eastern European
orphanages. *Clin Pediatr* 2003;42:585–90.

Budev MM, Arroliga AC, Falcone T. Ovarian hyperstimulation syndrome. *Crit
Care Med* 2005;33(suppl):S301–6.

Gunner MR, Bruce J, Grotevant HD. International adoption of institutionally
reared children: research and policy. *Dev Psychopathol* 2000;12:677–93.

Hansen M, Kurinczuk JJ, Bower C, Webb S. The risk of major birth defects
after intracytoplasmic sperm injection and in vitro fertilization. *N Engl J Med*
2002;346:725–30.

Heffner LJ. Advanced maternal age—how old is too old? *N Engl J Med* 2004;
351:1927–30.

Johnson DE. Long-term medical issues in international adoptees. *Pediatr Ann*
2000;29:234–41.

Joseph KS, Allen AC, Dodds L, et al. The perinatal effects of delayed child-
bearing. *Obstet Gynecol* 2005;105:1410–17.

Judge S. Developmental recovery and deficit in children adopted from Eastern
European orphanages. *Child Psychiatry Hum Dev* 2003;34:49–62.

Lambers DS, Clark KE. The maternal and fetal physiologic effects of nicotine.
Semin Perinatol 1996;20:115–26.

McGregor SG. A review of studies of the effect of severe malnutrition on mental development. *J Nutr* 1995;125:2233S–38S.

Miller LC, Kiernan MT, Mathers MI, Klein-Gitelman M. Developmental and
nutritional status of internationally adopted children. *Arch Pediatr Adolesc Med*
1995;140:40–44.

Nybo Andersen AM, Wohlfahrt J, Christens P, et al. Maternal age and fetal
loss: population based register linkage study. *BMJ* 2000;320:1708–12.

Papanikolaou EG, Pozzobon C, Kolibianakis EM, et al. Incidence and prediction
of ovarian hyperstimulation syndrome in women undergoing gonadotropin-
releasing hormone antagonist in vitro fertilization cycles. *Fertil Steril* 2006;
85:112–20.

Paulson RJ, Boostanfar R, Saadat P, et al. Pregnancy in the sixth decade of life:
obstetrical outcomes in women of advanced reproductive age. *JAMA* 2002;
28:2320–23.

Pharoah PO, Cooke T. Cerebral palsy and multiple births. *Arch Dis Child Fetal Neonatal Ed* 1996;75:F174.

Practice Committee of American Society for Reproductive Medicine. Smoking and infertility. *Fertil Steril* 2005;81:1181–86.

Quarles CS, Brodie J. Primary care of international adoptees. *Am Fam Physician* 1998;58:2025–32.

Rowe PJ, Comhaire FH, Hargreave TB, Mahmoud AMA. *WHO Manual for the Standardized Investigation, Diagnosis and Management of the Infertile Male.* Cambridge: Cambridge University Press, 2000.

Salihu HM, Shumpert MN, Slay M, et al. Childbearing beyond maternal age 50 and fetal outcomes in the United States. *Obstet Gynecol* 2003;102:1006–14.

Shiota K, Yamada S. Assisted reproductive technologies and birth defects. *Congenit Anom (Kyoto)* 2005;45:39–43.

Staat MA. Infectious disease issues in internationally adopted children. *Pediatr Infect Dis J* 2002;21:257–58.

Wood NS, Marlow N, Costelow K, et al. Neurologic and developmental disability after extremely preterm birth. *N Engl J Med* 2000;343:378–84.

Yokoyama Y. Prevalence of cerebral palsy in twins, triplets, and quadruplets. *Int J Epidemiol* 1995;24:943.

Chapter 12. Mental Health Risks for the Child

Barth RP, Crea TM, John K, et al. Beyond attachment theory and therapy: towards sensitive and evidence-based interventions with foster and adoptive families in distress. *Child Fam Soc Work* 2005;10:257–68.

Grantham-McGregor S. A review of studies of the effect of severe malnutrition on mental development. *J Nutr* 1995;125:2233S–38S.

Ingersoll BD. Psychiatric disorders among adopted children: a review and commentary. *Adoption Q* 1997;1:57–73.

International Consensus Statement on ADHD, January 2002. *Clin Child Fam Psychol Rev* 2002;5:89–111.

Johnson DE. Long-term medical issues in international adoptees. *Pediatr Ann* 2000;29:234–41.

Judge S. Developmental recovery and deficit in children adopted from Eastern European orphanages. *Child Psychiatry Hum Dev* 2003;34:49–62.

Juffer F, van Ijzendoorn MH. Behavior problems and mental health referrals of international adoptees: a meta analysis. *JAMA* 2005;293:2501–15.

Miller LC, Kiernan MT, Mathers MI, Klein-Gitelman M. Developmental and nutritional status of internationally adopted children. *Arch Pediatr Adolesc Med* 1995;140:40–44.

Chapter 13. Emotional Costs

adoption.com. Adoption Statistics (http://statistics.adoption.com).

Barth RP, Berry M. *Adoption and Disruption Rates, Risks, and Responses.* Hawthorne, NY: Aldine de Gruyter, 1988.

Ethics Committee of the American Society for Reproductive Medicine. Informing offspring of their conception by gamete donation. *Fertil Steril* 2004;81:527–31.

Evans MI, Goldberg JD, Gommergues M, et al. Efficacy of second-trimester selective termination for fetal abnormalities: international collaborative experience among the world's largest center. *Am J Obstet Gynecol* 1994;171:90–94.

Groze V. Special needs adoption. *Child Youth Serv Rev* 1986;8:363–73.

Groze V, Rosenberg K. *Clinical and Practice Issues in Adoption: Bridging the Gap between Adoptees Placed as Infants and as Older Children.* Westport, CT: Praeger, 1998.

Practice Committee of the American Society for Reproductive Medicine. Aging and infertility in women. *Fertil Steril* 2004;82:S102–5.

Ryan MA. *Ethics and Economics of Assisted Reproduction: The Cost of Longing.* Washington, DC: Georgetown University Press, 2001.

Stolley KS. Statistics on adoption in the United States. *The Future of Children: Adoption* 1993;3:26–42.

Chapter 14. Time Costs

American Adoptions. Adoption—How Long Is the Wait? (www.american adoptions.com/adopt/how_long).

Brown CA, Boone WR, Shapiro SS. Improved cryopreserved semen fecundability in an alternating fresh-frozen artificial insemination program. *Fertil Steril* 1988;50:825–27.

Byrd W, Drobnis EZ, Kutteh WH. Intrauterine insemination with frozen donor sperm: a prospective randomized trial comparing three different sperm preparation techniques. *Fertil Steril* 1994;62:850–56.

Centers for Disease Control and Prevention. 2003 Assisted Reproductive Technology (ART) Report: Section 1—Overview (data from the Society for Assisted Reproductive Technology) (www.cdc.gov/ART/ART2003/section1 .htm).

Centers for Disease Control and Prevention. 2004 Assisted Reproductive Technology (ART) Report (www.cdc.gov/ART/ART2004).

Chapter 17. Legal Considerations

Arizona Revised Statutes §28-218.

Arkansas Code §9-10-201.

Florida Statutes §63.042(3); §742.15.

Louisiana Revised Statutes §9:2713; §9:126 (1986).

Michigan Compiled Laws §722.855; §722.859; §722.861.

New York Consolidated Laws §121, *et seq.*

Texas Family Code §160.702; §160.754.

Washington Revised Code §26.26.230; §26.26.250.

INDEX

Page numbers in *italics* indicate figures and tables.